# Brave Hearts

# Brave Hearts

KEVIN WALTERS

IRONBARK
Pan Macmillan Australia

First published 1999 in Ironbark by Pan Macmillan Australia Pty Limited
St Martins Tower, 31 Market Street Sydney



National Library of Australia
cataloguing-in-publication data:

Walters, Kevin, 1967– .
Brave hearts.

ISBN 0 330 36182 1.

1. Walters, Kevin, 1967– . 2. Rugby League football players – Queensland – Biography. 3. Rugby League football players – Australia – Biography. 4. Breast – Cancer – Patients – Family relationships. I. Title.

796.3338092

Back cover photograph: Sportsphoto Agency and *Rugby League Week*
Typeset in 13/16pt New Baskerville by Post Pre-press Group
Printed in Australia by McPherson's Printing Group

# Contents

With Thanks vii

Foreword by Wayne Bennett 1

Introduction 5

CHAPTER ONE
IPSWICH BOY 7

CHAPTER TWO
CANE TOADS IN THE COLD 35

CHAPTER THREE
A HOT RECEPTION 48

CHAPTER FOUR
ORIGIN ANGST 64

CHAPTER FIVE
AS GOOD AS IT GETS 85

CHAPTER SIX
IN THE BRONCOS' STABLE 110

CHAPTER SEVEN
LOSING IT 138

CHAPTER EIGHT
LAUGHING AT LIFE 148

CHAPTER NINE
LOVE AND LOSS 166

CHAPTER TEN
KIM'S LEGACY 193

CHAPTER ELEVEN
HEART SONGS 202

CHAPTER TWELVE
FAREWELLS AND NEW HORIZONS 211

Afterwords 236

# WITH THANKS

This book couldn't have been written without the efforts and co-operation of the following people: my late wife Kim and our sons Jack, Billy and Jett; my mother and father, Sandra and Kevin Walters; and my brothers Kerrod, Steve, Andrew and Brett. Thanks to Kim's family also: Buddy, Rhonda and the Whole Facer gang, and Kim's mother Lorraine. Thank you Cara Weily and Narelle Bristow. Barry Collins, too. My gratitude goes to Wayne and Trish Bennett, Allan and Janine Langer, Chris Johns, Glenn Lazarus and all my football friends. I'm grateful to Larry Writer for his advice on how to put my thoughts and feelings into words. To Wally Lewis, Brad Fittler, Laurie Daley, Brad Izzard, Tony Durkin and Ben Elias, thanks for sharing your kind words with Damir Govorcin. David Middleton's excellent official rugby league yearbooks have been an invaluable reference source, as has the *Courier-Mail* of Brisbane and *Rugby League Week.* To Kathryn McKewin, Cherrell Hirst, Rebecca O'Gorman and Ray Crompton at the Wesley Hospital, thanks for establishing the Kim Walters Choices Program.

# FOREWORD

## *by Wayne Bennett*

Some people get excited driving to the Gold Coast, to MovieWorld or to the beach, but back in 1984 the most exciting trip a Brisbane football coach could have made was in the other direction, over to the playing fields of downtown Ipswich.

There a little fellow called Kevin Walters was just beginning to live out his big dreams, throwing footballs between his legs and around his back, charging to support his twin brother, Kerrod, like there was no tomorrow, and generally mesmerising the opposition. You talk about exciting.

Sure, they had bad habits and, equally sure, a lot to learn, which was soon realised when Kevin and Andrew, another Walters brother, arrived late for their first training session with the Queensland Under-18s.

They smiled, then frowned, blaming the train – an old red rattler – and I remember giving them a serve.

When I went south to coach Canberra in 1987

I took with me two guys: Peter Jackson and Kevin Walters. Kevvie had played Under-19s at Ipswich as well as some first grade, but he was ready and I took him.

Just a year later the Broncos were forming and I didn't want to go home without him. He still had two years to go on his contract and when I went to say I was sorry to be leaving he said not to worry, that he was happy in Canberra.

In 1990, his contract up, St George offered him $75,000 and the Broncos offered him $25,000 – Kevin Walters came home.

I know a little bit about the guy: I have seen him grow up, win five premierships, have been to his 21st, his engagement, his wedding, and to the funeral of his wife.

He represents everything you could want in a person, and in a friend. He is fun. Loyal. He speaks his mind. And he will never, ever let you down.

Often in life you hear people talking about 'family men'. Talk is cheap. Kevin Walters is a family man. Today, take one look at those three boys and the commitment he has made to them.

His parents, Sandy and Kevin (KG) – you just don't meet better people. You can see their character and their traits in all of the sons, but particularly Kevvie, who looks more like KG than KG himself.

People also talk about his great combination with Allan Langer, a combination borne out of friendship. In a decade of playing together they were partners in performance, and partners in mateship. Kevvie a great foil for Alf because he could read what Alf was going to do. If Alf was the heart and soul of the Broncos, Kevvie has been our emotion, a side to the guy that I love. He needs you to believe in him. And I do.

Back a couple of seasons now, he had a real thing about quitting the Broncos and moving to Townsville to play with the Cowboys. During it all, I went around and saw Kim, who, at that stage, didn't know whether she was going to get through her battle with breast cancer. Kim opened the door and smiled. 'Kim, he doesn't understand,' I said. 'The worst thing that can happen to you and to him now is to leave here, leave the support.' Kim said she appreciated that, and knew it was right. Kevvie? He never knew about the visit.

Going into that 1997 season, we were off to Papua New Guinea for a trial match and the night before Kevvie, all fired up, rang to say he wasn't going to New Guinea, that he wasn't doing this and he wasn't doing that and the Broncos could, well, take a hike.

The following morning I got to the airport early and found the seat where I could best look down the corridor at the passengers flowing in. I had never sat and looked down a corridor before, and I seemed to be doing it for a very long time. All of a sudden in he walked.

We won the Super League premiership that year, and the NRL premiership the following year, with Kevvie leading the way and playing for Australia.

He set up the Kim Walters Choices Program with the drive and commitment we have come to expect.

The emotion, too. In 16 years I have seen this young man go through everything, and come out the same.

Never have I felt more proud of a guy than when Kevin Walters led Queensland out of the tunnel in front of 90,000-odd screaming fans at Stadium Australia for the second game of the 1999 Origin series. Pride and emotion. It was the highlight – the salute – to everything he has done.

Wayne Bennett
June 1999

# INTRODUCTION

Until my wife Kim was diagnosed with breast cancer in August 1996, life for me was like a 30-metre sprint to the line with the fullback beaten and the crowd cheering. I was blessed. My family was large and loving. Kim, our sons Jack and Billy, and I lived in a sprawling ranch-style home set in hectares of green at Brookfield, west of Brisbane. Mum and Dad, my four brothers, Kim's family, and wonderful friends like Alf Langer, Wayne Bennett, Glenn Lazarus, Chris Johns and Peter Jackson made life rich. All that would be enough for any man. But, unlike any man, I had also toured twice with the Kangaroos, played 11 Tests for Australia, won 5 premierships and 22 State of Origins and, as five-eighth for the Broncos, was a member of rugby league's most lethal backline.

In 1993 I was quizzed by a reporter for one of those

magazine fact file features. The snappy revelations I reeled off included the fact that my name is Kevin David Walters, born on 20 October 1967 in Rockhampton. I revealed that I drove a Falcon S Pack, loved tennis and golf, considered Peter Jackson my favourite comedian, hung out at Daniel's Steakhouse and City Rowers nightclub, and in my next life wouldn't mind coming back as the world's No. 1 ranked tennis player. I grew serious, though, when the reporter asked me my idea of the ideal woman. 'I married her,' I said. My favourite relaxation? 'Spending time with my wife Kim and son Jack' (Billy and Jett hadn't been born then). When he asked me what I would be doing ten years from now, I didn't hesitate. 'Hopefully coaching somewhere, and helping Kim look after our four kids.' It was no fantasy; that was the future Kimmie and I had mapped out for ourselves. Life was good. Then, like an opponent who looms from a blind spot to crash-tackle you just as you're about to plant the ball over the tryline, fate, in the terrible and lethal form of Kim's cancer, tore my life apart.

This book is my story: Kevin Walters – son, brother, husband, father and footballer. It is also the story of Kim, the love of my life and mother of our sons, who adored and inspired us when she was alive and who continues, through our memories of the times we shared and the Kim Walters Choices Program, a cancer counselling service established in her name, to be a huge part of our lives even though she is gone.

CHAPTER ONE

# IPSWICH BOY

My mother Sandra – we often call her Sandy – and father Kevin – or KG – were both raised in Rockhampton, in Queensland. They were married in Rocky, too, but when Mum's father landed a job as station master at Ipswich railway station she wanted to stay close to her parents, so she and Dad came down as well. Within five years of being married, Sandy and KG had five sons – Brett, who's now (mid-1999) 36, Steve, 34, Andrew, 33, and me and my twin, Kerrod. We're 32, but Kerrod, super-competitive Kerrod, beat me into the world by fifteen minutes. Mum's a nurse, but the demands of caring for five hyperactive kids meant she couldn't work full-time. Dad is a carpenter and we all learned the trade too. The only trouble is, the houses my brothers build stay up while mine fall over.

We lived at 3 Merton Street near the railway line in

an old Queenslander house up on stumps. There were chooks down the back and it was the kids' job to collect the eggs. Kerrod and I shared a bedroom, so did Steve and Andrew, but Brett, the eldest son, had his own room. Underneath the house, the ground had been concreted so we could play cricket or ride our bikes in the shade away from the blazing subtropical sun. There was a corner where Dad had his workroom, always littered with tools and timber. Out the front, there was a fair-sized lawn, bisected straight down the middle by a concrete path.

Ipswich in the 1960s and 1970s was – as it remains today – a working-class town. Coal mining was the main industry, and many miners lived there. The railway was another big employer. Ipswich gets a bad rap from time to time as a rough place, but for the Walters kids, growing up there was fantastic. It's a sporting town. People love their sport at Ipswich – whether it be rugby league or union, cricket, soccer, baseball, tennis. Sport kept us off the streets, kept us away from drugs. As a boy I knew nothing about them. Of course, I smoked – we used to steal a few cigarettes from Dad – but that was it.

Dad was loving and kind, but he was a disciplinarian. My brothers and I were always getting strapped on the arse. When he caught us doing wrong he'd make us go to his and Mum's bedroom and take out his belt. Often we were punished in job lots. Dad would line up the five of us, make us pull our strides down, and *swish!* As strict as he was, though, his heart was not in corporal punishment and his beltings, while noisy, were pretty harmless. More for show than effect. Once, he gave Andrew, Kerrod and me the strap and we all ran to our rooms, but when Kerrod thought he was safe he started to laugh. 'Dad missed me!' he hooted. Unfortunately for Kerrod, Dad was passing by his room right then and heard him gleefully big-noting about how he had escaped unscathed. So Dad burst in and hauled Kerrod out and this time he didn't miss him. We all laugh about it today. None of us more than Dad. He's a funny man. He's not a guy who gets up on stage and makes people laugh, but if you're around him his humour is infectious. He can still break me up. Brother Steve is a very witty guy, and I'm sure he inherited his sense of humour from Dad and Mum. We've never thought twice about geeing each other up and playing practical jokes. Even as adults my brothers and I call our parents on the phone and pretend we're each other or a journo wanting to know why one or the other's form is lousy.

In my case the annoying habit started early. I'll let Mum go on with the story: 'I've worked in a nursing home a few days a week for 25 years, and when I first started little Kevvie was always ringing me up when I was flat out, wanting to know where his underpants or comb were. The other girls thought it was so funny. Then one day the phone rang when I was at work and it was for me. But all I could hear was this terrible heavy breathing on the other end of the line. Then a gruff voice said, "I've kidnapped your son, Kevin. If you want me to let him go you'll have to pay me money!" For a moment I was taken in, and then I realised it was Kevvie trying to extort some pocket money. So I said, "Oh, that's OK, keep him. You can have Kevin for nothing!" Well, you should have heard him get upset!'

Sandy had an abundance of love which she shared around her troublesome sons. As a small child I suffered from bad tonsillitis and it was like having my own nurse in the home. She once told a friend: 'He'd wake up at one or two o'clock in the morning with a high fever and I'd put him in the bath to get his temperature down. Next day he wouldn't be able to go to school and he'd sit around chewing gum because he'd be too sore to eat, and he'd play games of Monopoly against himself.'

Mum's sense of humour helped too. When Kerrod and his wife Maureen had their son Brooke in 1996, she took one look at the baby and remarked that he already had more hair than his father, whose locks were deserting him fast. And Brooke's big hands, she noted, would make him a natural golfer, which would suit his father who could caddy for him and snaffle a share of the prizemoney.

After that first glance at Brooke, she looked at him sleeping peacefully in his cot and said: 'When you see a little baby lying there a few hours old, so perfectly put together and so healthy, you realise how insignificant something like football really is.' But she was always there for us as kids, tending our footy wounds and cleaning our gear, encouraging us to play but never forcing us. In 1992, when we were all selected in the World Cup squad, she recalled to someone: 'They used to tell me all the time that they would become professional footballers.' She added, probably with a wry grin: 'They'd be in the yard playing after school, and I'd call them in to do their homework. I'd say, "You won't get through life playing football!"'

For all her protesting, Sandy relished the role of footy mum. Sandy is today a doting grandmother of 11 kids.

Like her, Dad was as supportive to us all as a parent could ever be. He took a big interest in our schooling, but knew in his heart that sport would always be more important to us than lessons. When we got into sport, he endlessly taxied us around the local cricket and footy fields. He and Mum devoted their weekends to making sure we all made our matches on time with our gear packed. Mum said later that if she'd not followed us around she'd have never seen us or Dad. My parents could have spent their weekends hanging out with their own friends or going away to the coast, but they sacrificed all that for us.

The Booval Swifts junior rugby league club was just 100 metres down our road, and it was there that we learned the skills of football. But it was in our yard that we learned to *compete.* We Walters boys were no different to Australian kids everywhere who turn a yard into a sporting arena. Those roughhouse, no-holds-barred family footy battles on our lawn – with oranges from the tree as halftime refreshment – were ideal training for the brutal Tests and State of Origin matches to come! I was always Tommy Raudonikis or Tommy Bishop. They were tough, scrappy halfbacks, even though Raudonikis was from New South Wales and Bishop was a Pom. Brett would be Bob Fulton, Steven was always Rod Reddy, Kerrod pretended to be the Manly enforcer Terry Randall, and Andrew, who followed Canterbury, was Terry Lamb.

But for all my wanting to play the hard man, I have to confess that I was a total sook. I was always in tears and throwing tantrums if the game didn't go my way or my brothers dished me out a bit of my own medicine. And if I was getting flogged as Tommy Raudonikis I'd suddenly transform into Tommy Bishop. Steve reckons I was the kind of kid who would cry if I couldn't throw a six in Monopoly. The cause of many of my problems was the concrete path that bisected the yard. Mum and Dad, who refereed our games, pulling us up for claiming unfair tries and making high tackles, insisted that the dreaded path was out of bounds. They were scared, and quite reasonably so, that we would break bones or crack heads on it. We loved hurling each other onto the concrete when games got heated, and they always did. Tackling your brother or one of the other neighbourhood kids on the concrete brought an automatic penalty or the sin bin. Mum invented the bin long before anyone else thought of it, and it was usually occupied by one of us. Out-of-control biffo was the signal for Mum to resort to the garden hose. A blast of water was guaranteed to cool the combatants down.

All our lives centred on those bloodcurdling contests. When mobile phones came in, Dad was a big fan and snapped one up immediately. Having a mobile meant that he could call Mum on his way home from work. 'Sandy,' he'd say, 'I'm 20 minutes from home. Throw the stubbies in the freezer!' The sight of Dad sitting on the step drinking his half-dozen stubbies and puffing away on his smokes while trying to enforce the rules as we played until dark will stay with me forever. So will the memory of the thrill we got when, to commemorate floodlights being erected at Lang Park, he set up his own light in the yard so we, too, could play night football.

Sometimes our games were simply excuses to beat each other up. We brothers have always loved to rumble with each other. Nothing malicious, because we've always been great mates, just very physical sibling rivalry. We were only kids trying to be tough, I suppose; standing up for ourselves. Kerrod was the only one of us who wasn't keen on biffo and took little part in brotherly assault and battery. Funny how he ended up with the worst football judiciary record! Andrew, a mad redhead, and I would get stuck into each other like cats and dogs. And I didn't mind sledging the older and stronger Steve. I used to tell him I was running at him because he couldn't tackle. But the sledging was all in fun. We were always close in spite of everything and, if an outsider picked on any of us, then he had all the brothers to contend with. If anything, we're closer now that we're older – and of course we don't bash each other up any more. Well, not as often, anyway.

When we played together, Kerrod and I worked up a good combination. Being twins gave us an almost telepathic understanding of what each other was doing on the field. Always playing on the same team in backyard footy paid off in the big-time, too. In one early game, for Ipswich against Redcliffe, everything we did turned to gold. All our plays in the yard at home came off and that was a bloody good feeling. I always liked playing with my brothers. I think I'm the only one of the five who has played with each of the others. That's something I've got on all of them, isn't it!

Andrew, or 'Drew', was a prop and second rower who could have gone as far in the game as Kerrod, Steve and me, but he was badly injured in an Under-18 match. In a simple tackle he displaced the vertebrae in his neck and had to have intensive surgery, which included a bone graft. Mum and Dad were devastated, but for all their deep worry they never tried to stop us playing rugby league. 'There were people who couldn't believe that Sandra and I could allow the kid to play again after such an injury,' said Dad later, 'but it was his life.' Drew's neck injury sidelined him for two years. Dad recalled: 'He moped around the house and never took an interest in anything. The other boys would be off playing and Andrew wasn't even interested in watching them. Without footy, his whole personality changed, he missed it so much. It wasn't our decision for him to play again. We all agreed we would go along with what the specialist said, and agreed he could play as long as it wasn't at hooker.' In the end the whole family accepted that in any contact sport there would be accidents but that the joy of playing far outweighed the risk. Drew made a comeback, but by then he had lost a little of his interest and passion for rugby league. Many good judges who saw him play as a junior say he could have ended up a better player than any of us. He was offered a contract by Canberra in the mid-1980s but knocked it back. Then he joined the Broncos but never recovered the form of his younger days.

Andrew was a redhead in a family of brown-haired kids, so we gave it to him about that. Our sledging about his hair got to him so bad that Drew was asking Mum to show him his adoption certificate. Our brother Brett copped it because he wasn't as good as the rest of us at catching the football, although he was big, strong and fast. I always thought Steve was the apple of Mum and Dad's eye. Parents don't like to admit it but sometimes they have favourites, and Steve used to grab Mum's hair and pull it and say: 'Who's your favourite son?' He wouldn't let go until she told him it was him. Steve was the brainiest of us all. He was a top cricketer, too. He went to Ipswich Grammar with Craig McDermott, who grew up to become one of Australia's finest fast bowlers. Steve's claim to fame is that he took more wickets than Craig in the final year of school and pipped him to be named Grammar's Sportsman of the Year for his footy, cricket, tennis and swimming feats. He never took cricket too seriously. When he'd come to bowl, the umpire would ask him, 'What do you bowl, son?' and he'd reply, 'Right-arm trash.'

Steve has just wound up his long career this year, 1999, with the Newcastle Knights, after playing for 11 years at Canberra and a season at North Queensland, along with 14 State of Origin matches and 15 Tests. He was one of the best – if not *the* best – hooker forwards of all time. Hookers don't like giving their rivals a wrap, so it meant a lot when Penrith's great rake Royce Simmons said of Steve in 1996: 'No doubt . . . Steve is the best there's been. His service out of dummy half is superb. He can snap a pass straight off the ground both ways. He can pass long, too, and is smart enough to keep markers off the ball runners. He's real quick out of dummy half and knows when to run. He can steer his forwards around the field. His work-rate is high. His defence is great and he's a tough coot. He locks the ball up in tackles. Geez, you couldn't be much more complete.'

And John Lang, a former Test hooker and now coach of the Sharks, remembers young Steve in the mid-1980s: 'We realised then that Steve was going to be a great player. The only doubt we had about him was that he was too good-looking for a hooker – but he seems to have overcome that problem.'

Kerrod, who played a decade of seasons for the Broncos, six Origin games and eight Tests, and after a season with Adelaide is finishing his career at the English club, Gateshead, was just as good a hooker as Steve, but he was singled out by the judiciary a fair bit and controversial suspensions for punching and high tackles dinted his confidence. In 1989 and 1990 he'd be chosen in the rep teams before Steve – Kerrod and I made the 1990 Kangaroos; Steve was overlooked – but Steve got the jump on Kerrod in the early 1990s and never looked back. There was a terrific highlight when Kerrod, Steve and I were all selected in the 1992 World Cup team to England. The family skimped and saved to come over, and on the day we played Great Britain in that memorable World Cup final the stands of Wembley Stadium were full of Walters! Steve won the Player of the Match and I set up the winning try for Steve Renouf in our narrow 10–6 victory. A magic memory, just magic! It's such a buzz that brother Steve, Kerrod and I have reached the levels in the game that we have. No other family has supplied three brothers who've played for Australia.

Just as the fur flew in the yard at home when Kerrod and I and Steve lined up against each other, there were often fireworks when we played against each other in first grade. 'Like a lot of players in the competition, I'd love to drop Kevin on his backside,' Steve once said. 'Only trouble is, I can't catch him.' He *did* catch up with Kerrod one day at Bruce Stadium. Steve elbowed Kerrod in the head and gave him a cauliflower ear. 'He reckons it was an accident,' said Kerrod at the time, nursing his throbbing lug, 'but Mum wasn't too happy about it.' Broncos coach Wayne Bennett was furious with Steve and said he was going to cite him, but I'm not sure how serious he was about that. Mum and Dad were ropable. My brothers laughed about the incident around the dinner table, but each took his football deadly seriously – and deep down we are all as competitive as any player I've ever known. I never enjoy playing against my brothers, because I know there is little room for brotherly love on the field. After I went to play for the Canberra Raiders in 1987, leaving Kerrod to become a Bronco alone, Mum would remark: 'I was really wild to see the twins split up. It didn't seem right.'

I have been in Broncos team meetings before a game against Canberra, North Queensland, Adelaide or Newcastle, when we'd be working out a strategy to get over the top of our opponents and Steve and Kerrod's name would come up. Someone would say: 'We've gotta belt that Walters! Let's get stuck into 'im.' When that happened I felt like standing up and saying: 'Leave him alone, you bastard!' It would upset me to hear the boys talk about my brothers like that. I could never help myself. If anyone ever belted Kerrod or Steve on the field, they'd have to deal with me too. I even felt bad if the Broncos were putting the cleaners through one of my brothers' *teams.* I remember walking back to halfway after we'd scored another try in a flogging of North Queensland, feeling really sorry for Steve. You're not supposed to feel sorry for the opposition in rugby league. Dad and Mum are the same. Dad once said that he hated it when we played against each other.

KG and Sandy were careful never to play favourites, even going to the extreme length of wearing Broncos *and* Raiders clothing on match days. Mum remembers: 'Kevin was always checking me out before we set off for the ground to make sure I wasn't wearing any of the other team's colours. "What about that green handkerchief?" he'd say. It was shocking when Brisbane played Canberra. I really hated the boys being up against each other. Steve used to ring Kerrod and Kevin before the game and tell them to be sure to wear their helmets in the game because he was gonna get them. Then Stevie would do something good in the match and I'd cheer and then I'd stop myself because I realised by cheering for Steve I was cheering against the Broncos, and vice versa. Sometimes I wouldn't even go to the game. Oh, I couldn't bear it.'

When I was starting out in first grade, Kerrod was my inspiration. I was proud that he was a regular Queensland Origin player in 1989 when I was struggling to make first grade at Canberra. Kerrod played all three Tests against the Kiwis that year as well. I got a lot of motivation from his achievements.

Steve is also close to me in temperament. Steve is a joker and loves a laugh. A very witty guy. He is also switched on financially and has made some good business decisions over the years. He has two kids. Steve was determined to end his career on a high, and didn't enjoy his year at North Queensland when he was in and out of first grade. He says he enjoyed playing his final season at Newcastle, packing down between Paul Harragon (until the Chief retired in May) and Anthony Butterfield. He wanted to go to a club where he thought he had a chance of winning a premiership or at least winning more games than you lose. The Johns boys tried to teach him how to surf, but they had their work cut out because Steve is no wave-rider. There are no surf clubs in Ipswich!

Both my brothers have been affected in their final years in the game by the trend to play halfbacks and five-eighths at hooker. In Steve and Kerrod's heyday, hooker was a specialist position. Tough, smart scrummagers that were specialist organising dummy halves who kept up momentum in attack were prized players in our game. Today, the 10-metre ruck rule means that hookers must be speedsters who can scoot forward after a quick play-the-ball to keep a roll-on. Once, hookers competed against their opposite number for the ball. Scrums were a contest where anything went. No more. About the only advantage an old-style hooker has over a converted back in the modern game is his ability to carry out the heavy, middle-of-the-ruck defence. Kerrod found, when the Adelaide Rams folded at the end of the 1998 season, that he had to go to England to get a game. He hooked up there with a new Super League franchise, Gateshead. Other Australians are playing there and the coach is Shaun McRae, who was a trainer at Canberra and for the Kangaroos in 1990 and 1994, coached at St Helens and was co-coach of the British Test side. Kerrod returned home midway through season 1999 after his wife Maureen, who had remained in Australia with their four-year-old son, Brooke, suffered head injuries in a bus accident while on holidays in Asia. Kerrod took leave of absence from Gateshead and rushed home to be with his family. Maureen is now making a good recovery and Kerrod is back in England.

Brett and Drew, for any number of reasons, didn't represent their country, but they both played for Queensland junior teams and were solid first graders.

These days, Brett toils away as a carpenter. He has been married twice and it's a big family joke that he can't walk past a church without going in and getting hitched. Every time he passes a church we *grab* him so he doesn't go in and whisk some woman up to the altar. He has been through some rough personal times, but now leads a calm, laid-back lifestyle with nothing worrying him these days. He and Drew were in a carpentry business together but Drew's now working at the Jacaranda milk factory in Ipswich. When Drew told his kids he had a job there, they were over the moon. His boy Josh went to school and boasted: 'My Dad works at the milk factory and he can drink *any* flavour milk he wants *any time*!' Drew's always been a bit of a battler, he doesn't live in a mansion, but he's content with his life and that puts him way ahead of many people, in my view.

We're a close family today and have no trouble expressing our affection for each other. We see each other whenever we can. But back when we were kids, it was often Kerrod and me against the rest. Because we were twins and the youngest, we were inseparable. Mum would tell people: 'In their games out in the yard the twins used to get a terrible flogging from the bigger boys, but they always came back for more. It was there they learnt what being competitive was all about.' When Steve and Brett were in their early teens and beginning to notice girls, and Kerrod and I were still about 10, they'd give us the brush-off. They'd yell: 'Scram, you're too little!' We didn't mind, because we hated girls and, besides, we had a ton of fun knocking around together. Wherever he went, I went; and wherever I went, he went.

We both joined Booval Swifts in 1974 and played together in the Under-7s. One memorable day, when Andrew's Under-8 team had some injuries, we were promoted to play on the wings to make up the numbers in the higher division. Our opponents were North Ipswich. They had a tiny blond halfback who got the ball, ran around our entire team and scored. After the match, Kerrod says today, he went up to shake young Allan Langer's hand and said: 'Matey, if you can run around me like that you're going to play for Australia one day.'

Ipswich being a sporting town and not a large one in those days, the paths of the Walters family and the Langers – Allan, his father Harry, mother Rita, sister Desley and brothers Cliff, Kevin and Neville – crossed repeatedly. Allan and Drew played against each other for Norths and Booval Swifts in the age group ahead of Kerrod and me. My brother Steve and Neville Langer, who are the same age, played against each other and joined up in the Ipswich rep team together year after year. Brother Brett and Kevin Langer were contemporaries. Inevitably, the Langers and the Walters became close. Our dad and Alf's father Harry, who was a carriage builder for Queensland Railways, had a bit to do with our teams and occasionally after work they would meet over a few beers under our house while we kids took on each other in backyard football. It was there, I suppose, under my dad's makeshift floodlight, that Alf's and my future intuitive combination for the Broncos, Queensland and Australia kicked off. Today, Alf Langer, a funny, good-hearted man and a fabulous rugby league player until his shock retirement midway through the 1999 season, remains my close friend.

One day when I was about 15 I got the surprise of my life. There was a knock on the door and standing there was Tommy Raudonikis – the *real* Tommy Raudonikis. When the former Western Suburbs, NSW and Australian halfback star was booted out as coach of Brothers in 1985 after he got involved in a pub brawl when he stuck up for a player who was copping a belting, he was made coach of the senior Ipswich team, the Ipswich Jets, who played in the Queensland State League. He told Dad that he'd spotted Kerrod and me playing for Booval Swifts and wanted us with him at the Jets the following year. I couldn't believe it! Tom Raudonikis at *our* house! About a month later we played a game against another junior team, and there was Tom, in his 40s and long retired as a player, feeding the scrum for them. He saw these other guys getting flogged by us and just pulled on a pair of boots to lend them a hand. Kerrod and I had spent all those years watching Tommy on TV and pretending to be him in our backyard, and here he was on the other team. Even if I could have, there was no way I was going to belt my old idol. He was way, way past his best, but even then his competitiveness was unbelievable. Unfortunately, when we joined the Ipswich Jets Kerrod and I were still young and played most of our footy with them in the Under-19s. Tom coached firsts and we were only picked in the top grade four or five times, so his influence on us wasn't great. I do remember some of his fire-and-brimstone speeches to his players, though, and learned that he nailed a raw bullock's heart to the dressing room wall and made each player squeeze it – the idea being, I guess, that the fighting spirit of the bull was passed on to the player.

Kerrod and I attended Bremer State High up to Year 10, then finished our secondary education at Ipswich Grammar, the oldest grammar school in Queensland. They used to drum that into us: '1863, red and white.' The school was proud of its academic and sporting achievements, and as well as my brothers and me and Craig McDermott, Willie Carne and Craig Polla-Mounter went there. I was fine academically at Bremer, but in Years 11 and 12 at Ipswich Grammar sport outpointed schoolbooks and I lost the plot a little. 'Kevin could have been a better student,' Dick Rima, my maths teacher who is now deputy headmaster at Grammar, once said. He went on: 'But he was a good kid and well-behaved. His sense of humour certainly enlivened the class. He had a bit of the devil about him. If he'd studied harder he could have got better marks, because he was capable. In those days, he looked pretty much the same as now: chunky with a crewcut. He's got a few more muscles these days. After he left school and was making it as a big-time footballer he'd always say "Hi" when we met around Ipswich. The same old Kevin with a big smile on his face. His parents Kevin and Sandra were marvellous people.'

Dick and the other teachers at Ipswich Grammar could have been excused for having high hopes for Kerrod and me. Steve had been at the school before us and he had done well at maths, physics, chemistry and so on. The teachers may have expected more of the same from us, but how were they to know that, being twins, Kerrod and I had only half a brain each! The bottom line was that when we left the school my nickname was 'Thick' and Kerrod's was 'Brick'. Enough said.

We played rugby for Ipswich Grammar on Saturdays and league for Booval Swifts on Sundays. At Swifts we won the comp every year but one, from Under-7s to Under-18s. When we were at Ipswich, me at halfback and Kerrod in the centre, they won rugby union premierships they hadn't won for 50 years. It just goes to show that even if you don't have too many brains you can still contribute. I reckon I gave something back to the school in my own way. It was at Ipswich Grammar that we met Steve Nance, the physical education teacher there, who also trained the Ipswich Jets and went on to train the Broncos years later. Steve coached the school's Under-16A rugby side, which Kerrod and I were involved in, and also took us for PE. That was the part of the curriculum we thrived on. Sport was so well organised and a lot of our future success is due to what we learned from Steve Nance at Ipswich Grammar.

In one regard, Bremer High had it all over Ipswich Grammar. Bremer was co-ed. When I was there I was vaguely aware of a pretty blonde girl named Kim

Facer. I knew she was around – she was such a knockout you couldn't miss her – but I never really got to know her. That came later. She left Bremer in Year 10 and I went to Ipswich Grammar, and it wasn't until then, when we were 17, that friends introduced us. Kim's beauty and happy spirit knocked me sideways. I was impressed, which is putting it mildly, and I asked her to be my date at a ball to celebrate Ipswich Grammar First XV's premiership win. Kerrod's date that night was Maureen, who is now his wife. It was my first date, and I'm sure it was his too.

It would be nice to tell you how Kim and I fell in love and were together from then on, but that's not quite the way it was. We went out together for a few months, then she got her driver's licence and she motored out of my life for a while. She ditched me for a 1972 Ford Escort. That's what bugged me more than anything: it was such a beat-up old car, and for a while there she loved it more than me! After she gave me the flick pass for a couple of months, she took me back. We fell in love and that was it. I loved her from our first year together and have never stopped loving her. Mum and Dad thought she was great. To Mum, Kim was the daughter she'd never had. The remarkable thing about Kim – one of so many remarkable things about her – was that somehow she grew more beautiful as she got older. As a girl growing up in Toowoomba, she won local beauty and charity pageants and was Toowoomba's Queen of Flowers and Maid of Honour. Some women are great beauties when young and their looks fade with the years and increasing responsibilities, and having children. Not Kim. In my eyes, anyway, she became more gorgeous with every new year. In her late 20s she was a total stunner, and then, of course, her cancer began to take its toll.

As well as good looks, Kim was smart, loved a good time and had a strong and gutsy character. About the only downside to Kim was her ferociously protective father. Buddy Facer was a local terror. Everyone had heard of Buddy. He was a wild man. He was a boxer, and not all of his fights were in the ring. He was – how can I put it? – larger than life. Buddy used to cause the odd problem for the constabulary, and one cop with whom he'd had a few run-ins was a young bloke who'd played on the wing for Australia and, since retiring as a player, was making a name for himself as a coach. His name was Wayne Bennett. One night, after Buddy had got to know me and trust me with Kim, we were having a drink together in the den at Buddy's house when the phone rang. It was Wayne, looking for me. He wanted to talk to me about footy and my parents had given him Buddy's number.

'Hello, Buddy Facer,' said Buddy. 'Yeah, Kevvie's here. Who wants him?' When Wayne told him who it was, Buddy nearly fell off his chair. 'Wayne Bennett! You're kidding! Are you sure this is Wayne Bennett? And it's not *me* you're after? It's *Kevin*?' Buddy was relieved and impressed at the company I kept. And when Wayne finally met Kim he couldn't believe what a small world it is. Here's me going out with the notorious Buddy's beautiful daughter. '*You* taking *Buddy*

*Facer*'s daughter out!' said Wayne in disbelief. 'He'll kill you!' In time, Wayne and Buddy became good friends, and Wayne was there for Buddy when tragedy struck later.

Early on, I was shit-scared of Buddy. It was always: 'Yes, sir. No, sir.' He was a very intimidating man. I had a rattly old Mazda and when I would pay a secret call to Kim late at night I used to turn the lights and the motor off and try to roll silently down the hill to her house. Kim's bedroom was downstairs and I used to get out of the car and race into the Facers' house and into Kim's room. I was certain I was putting one over Buddy and that he had no idea about our rendezvous. Years later he told me he was up to speed with everything and, in spite of being as protective as a pitbull of Kim, he approved because he knew ours was a love that would last. How right he was. Buddy says today about those times: 'I'd always hear Kevin sneak down the hill to our place in his Mazda. He didn't know that, and he didn't know I'd hear him sneak back up the hill in the morning. I knew what they were up to all along, but although I was a strict father I didn't really mind because I knew they were right for each other. Kim knew from the first that Kevin was the man for her, and what was good enough for Kim was good enough for me. He was a good young bloke and he came from a wonderful family. KG and Sandy were always friendly to us and offered a bed and food to any friend who wanted to sleep over. I had a room at my house I called the dungeon. Only two or three weeks after Kevin started taking Kim out, he'd pull up and come straight to the dungeon to have a drink with me. Kim would complain: "Dad, Kevin's spending more time in here with you than he is with me!'"

As Buddy says, he and I have been friends from the start. I've always respected him and I know he respects me and loves my sons, Jack, Billy and Jett. Even though our beloved Kim is no longer with us, our friendship continues and we'll be mates for life.

Kim's mother is Lorraine. She and Buddy split up at about the time I met Kim and she went to live on the Gold Coast. Today we ring each other every week and she sees the boys regularly. She was always very supportive of Kim and me. Buddy's wife, Rhonda, has been wonderful as well. Kim's sister Kelly (her nickname is 'Rach') and Kim were always close, even though Kim was 11 years older. When Buddy and Lorraine broke up, Kelly lived with her mum. Kelly moved in with us to help out when Kim got sick in 1996, and was a tower of strength.

Kim and I got up to the things all young lovers do. I can't say I ever treated Kim to the deep-fried delights on offer at Pauline Hanson's fish and chip shop (I had never heard of her until the last couple of years), but we went out on Friday and Saturday nights with my brothers and their girlfriends and all our friends to pubs, each other's houses, or clubs like Caesar's Palace and the Roman Lounge, whose names were a whole lot more swish than the joints themselves. Alf Langer and his girlfriend Janine, now his wife, were hanging out with us by then. Buddy Facer remembers Alf, when he worked for Ipswich Council, always coming out and cleaning up the area around Buddy and Kim's house after a storm. Buddy got first-cab-off-the-rank treatment because of our friendship. It may have been an extension of our backyard football battle-royals when the Langer brothers would join in, but on our nights out Alf and I began to perfect our party trick that has alarmed bystanders from Ipswich to Manchester. We have this talent for staging fake but very realistic fights. Alf can fall down without hurting himself and I toss him into walls and garbage bins, down stairs, into the gutter – really giving him a going over. He'll lie there in a heap as if unconscious and just when people are thinking they'd better call an ambulance, he'll give a big wink and jump to his feet completely unscathed. Once on the 1990 Kangaroo tour in the north of England after a night at a pub we put on such a blue that English bruisers wanted to tear me apart for beating up the little blond chap. We'd get right into it, and although we'd never get hurt our clothes were often ripped and tattered after a night out.

Ipswich gets a bad rap from time to time, but I enjoyed growing up there. I'm more than happy to say that I come from Ipswich. People often call Ipswich 'Two-Head City,' but every town has its problems. From our experience, Ipswich is a good place to bring up children. The houses may not be as expensive as in Brisbane, and it is definitely working class, but the people here are no different from anywhere else. Mum and Dad still live in Merton Street. Unfortunately, as I had moved away at the age of 19, I lost contact with a lot of friends. Today I visit every chance

I get. My son Jack plays with Booval Swifts Under-8s and we have a lamb roast with Mum and Dad after his training on Wednesday nights. We're a tight and close-knit family. Family values are so important. I think they've been swept aside in today's society. Simple things like sitting down at the table and having a family meal together. I'll be forever in my family's debt for all they've done for us through Kim's illness and her death in 1998. They would have done it for any of us brothers, but they've supported me 100 per cent. It's so comforting to know that you've got people in your corner who love you and care for you, and I feel the same way about them. The biggest compliment I can pay Sandy and KG is that I'm going to bring my boys up the way they raised me.

Ipswich is a real rugby league town. When Ipswich played Toowoomba at the local oval there would be huge crowds and the game was a real social event. In the late 1950s and early 1960s the Australian front row – Gary Parcell, Noel Kelly and Dud Beattie – were Ipswich lads. We used to call Beattie 'Uncle Dud' when he became a Queensland and Australian selector. If there was an Ipswich guy competing for a rep position with a bloke from somewhere else, the Ipswich player would always get Uncle Dud's vote.

When I was 13, I was one of 31,000 people sardined into Lang Park on 8 July 1980 for that legendary first State of Origin match, when Queensland's 35-year-old captain Arthur Beetson whacked his Parramatta teammate and good friend Mick Cronin, the NSW centre, and set the blood-and-guts precedent for this fabulous contest. My memory is a bit hazy, but I think perhaps the Langer kids were with us too that night. Dad loaded us all into his yellow Kingswood station wagon for the drive to Lang Park. When we got there the streets all around were packed with people trying to get in. We were standing in a long queue and Dad said to us: 'Look, I don't think we're gonna get in.' So I started bawling and howling: 'Ohh, I wanna go to the game!' Dad has always had trouble refusing me, so he said, 'Stay here', and strolled down to the front of the queue, did a quick sidestep into the crowd at the ticket office and a few minutes later returned with tickets for us all. We thought he was the best thing since sliced bread.

Getting a seat was extra important to us because Brett was playing in the Under-18 curtain raiser. I remember Beetso belting the Crow right in front of us, *whack!*, and Craig Young covered in blood. Queensland won 20–10. I thought how good would it be to be out there in the maroon jumper doing what these blokes were doing to the Blues, who'd been thrashing Queensland for as long as any of us could remember. A long-haired Wally Lewis locked the Maroons' scrum that night. Wally was such a hero to me, and I was ashamed when he came to play against Ipswich in a State Cup game and a cage-type structure had to be set up to protect him from crowd abuse because the locals resented him for being such a great player. Why do we treat our sporting champions so badly? In America they honour sporting stars as heroes, but here we seem to want to knock them down. Even Alf at various times in his career was hated outside Brisbane. In the early 1990s, *Inside Sport* magazine ran a poll and Alf got the vote as the most hated sportsman in Australia. I don't know why; maybe people are just jealous.

In 1984 and 1985, Alf, Drew and I played in the Queensland Under-18 and Under-19 teams, coached by Wayne Bennett, who was then in charge of Brisbane Souths. I got a start in the 1984 State side after Alf hurt his ankle in a trial. We were all carefree young blokes, not really into discipline, and didn't know what we were in for with the stern and scary coach. Andrew and I found out soon enough. We were at a training camp up at Maroochydore Surf Lifesaving Club. We arrived five minutes late for an 11 a.m. team meeting and Wayne hauled us over the coals in front of all the other blokes. 'Who the hell do you think you are?' he raged at us. 'Not only are you holding me up, you're holding up your team-mates too. Show some respect, or piss off!' We were all thinking: 'Shit! This bloke's bloody fair dinkum.' I'd never seen anything so heavy in my life and I thought: 'Christ! I'm scared of this bloke. I'm gonna do the right thing.'

Wayne must have seen something to like about my play and when he was signed as coach of Canberra for the 1987 season, he asked me to join him there. Steve was already a Raider by then, after starting his career with Brisbane Norths, but I was a little hesitant to head south because Kerrod wasn't going and I wasn't sure how Kim would react to leaving Ipswich and her family for the cold and unfamiliar national capital. But when I put it to her, she said that wherever I went she was going too. Though we weren't married, Kim's mum and dad gave us their blessing. Buddy remarked later: 'They came to me about going to Canberra. There was no thinking to do, she was in good hands. I said, "Go for it."'

Kim raced off to pack our bags. I called Wayne and told him: 'I'm a Raider.'

CHAPTER TWO

# CANE TOADS IN THE COLD

Kim and I settled into Canberra life fairly easily. Of course, we missed our families and the town where we'd grown up. But it was an adventure and we threw ourselves into the new experience. If being given a nickname by team-mates is proof that you're accepted in the side, then I was highly honoured. At Canberra I had three nicknames: 'Splinters' because I spent so much time on the bench; 'Unit' because I was a tubby little bloke in those pre-nutrition-conscious days who gorged on every kind of junk food, drank and smoked a packet of cigarettes a day; and 'Toad' because I hailed from the land of the cane toad. Team-mate Rowan Brennan made it really personal after he read an article in *Australasian Post* magazine about a monster cane toad who'd migrated to New South Wales from Queensland. It had been christened 'Yuck' because it was so damned ugly. Rowan started calling me 'Yuck' and, of course, the name stuck for a while.

Kim and I found a place to live and were never lonely, making friends with my new team-mates and their partners. Steve of course, who was the Raiders' star hooker (and whose nickname was 'Boxhead'), looked after us and helped us settle into the new environment. Even then, Kim was crazy about kids. She was always clucky and didn't have to be asked twice to babysit the kids of the older players, such as Gary Coyne. She'd come home all glowing after being with the little ones. Having children of our own was not the furthest thing from our mind when we got engaged in 1988.

In 1987 the Raiders, jointly coached by Wayne Bennett and Test coach Don Furner, were still feeling their way. They were just five years old and still two years away from their first premiership win in that classic grand final against Balmain. The signs were there, though, in 1987 when we made the grand final and the next year too, that it was only a matter of time before Canberra made their mark on the premiership. Steve, Kiwi international Brent Todd, Dean Lance, Gary Coyne and Sam Backo were the nucleus of the pack, with the promising young Glenn Lazarus and Brad Clyde being blooded from the bench. In the backs there was the great Mal Meninga and Gary Belcher, both fresh from Brisbane Souths, Chris O'Sullivan, the mercurial winger John Ferguson, tearaway teenager Laurie Daley who would be an on-field rival and off-field friend throughout my career, and another bloke, a centre and five-eighth also from Brisbane Souths who was as funny as he was skilled with a football. His name was Peter Jackson, but to all of us he was 'Jacko' or 'Action' after the kids' hero Action Jackson.

The 1987 grand final was one big highlight of my Canberra years. The other was getting to know the unforgettable, hilarious, doomed Jacko. So many memories. He was a dashing, good-looking man, always smiling, clowning around, bumming cigarettes. He'd do anything for a laugh. He seemed the most unlikely bloke to suffer depression and die, aged only 33, in November 1997, after an apparent drug overdose. On the field, in the dressing room and the club, on radio and TV, Jacko's one-liners would break you up. He once said of himself: 'Some people are boring, and some ain't. I just try to make light of most things. That's just the way I am, although people can get the impression I'm not fair dinkum.' But he *was* fair dinkum.

As a player he was ruthless. Ask former South Sydney star Steve Mavin who was destroyed by Jacko's grubber-kick barrage in a semi-final. I played in that game and saw it for myself at close range. Steve, a fine player, could not handle the sustained pressure and his handling lapses let in Canberra tries. His confidence was ruined and his coach George Piggins hauled him out of the game. Steve was never really a force again. Never let anyone tell you rugby league is not a merciless game; it can chew you up and spit you out. I felt so sorry for Steve Mavin. Or ask the feared Penrith and Australian enforcer Mark 'MG' Geyer if Jacko was not fair dinkum. In Origin II in 1991, the game where MG and Wally Lewis almost came to blows at the halftime break, MG flattened Queensland fullback Paul Hauff with a high shot. Jacko saw red, and set off after MG, throwing plenty of punches. Mark towered over Jacko, but his own safety was the last thing on Peter's mind when he saw his team-mate felled. Or ask me if Jacko was fair dinkum. In 1988 I played alongside him in the centres against Balmain and he put me over for three tries. That year he was the best centre in the game. In coping with his illnesses, which included severe depression and, finally, heroin addiction, Jacko was *definitely* fair dinkum. But in the end courage and a quip were not enough.

I first came across Peter Jackson when I was playing for Ipswich against his club, South Brisbane. Jacko scooped up a handful of dirt and threw it in my face because he thought Kerrod and I were up-and-comers and he was a couple of years older and well established as an Origin player and wanted to show me who was boss. 'I'll give it to you, you little bastard,' he yelled at me. 'Comin' in here thinkin' you can do this 'n' do that!' I was ready to fight him, but his big grin won me over and we had a beer in the clubhouse after the game. Our coach Tom Raudonikis joined us and told Jacko he wanted to sign him for Ipswich. Tommy wrote his phone number on the back of a cigarette packet and gave it to Jacko, saying: 'Here, mate, take this, give us a ring – we could use you up here.' That was Tommy all over. And Jacko said to Tom: 'Well, you better buy me a carton of beer for the drive home, eh!' Tommy bought him a carton and I said: 'Jacko, you won't need all of those beers, mate, you're only driving to Brisbane!' He replied, quick as a flash: 'Well, you never know, I might get stuck in traffic.' Off he trotted with his bag over one arm and his carton of XXXX cans under the other. I thought: 'Jesus, I like this bloke!'

He played Origin for Queensland in 1986 and our friendship picked up at the Raiders in 1987. The following year he made his Test debut against Great Britain in the 100th Test match between the old enemies. Jacko scored two tries in Australia's 17–6 win. He quit Canberra at the end of 1988 to rejoin Wayne at the Broncos. We palled up again at Brisbane when I went north in 1990.

Though he was an established Queensland and Australian representative, Jacko had an unsettled two years with the Broncos. He upped stakes and headed south again in 1991 with his wife Siobhan and daughter Lucy to play out his career with North Sydney. We always bagged him because every time he left a club they won a premiership. He'd left Canberra in 1988 and they won in 1989, and when the Broncos carried off the comp in 1992 he'd left for North Sydney. He deserved to win a premiership. At the Bears in 1991 and 1992, he again played for Australia. He retired from the game in 1993 to do what everyone always knew he would: become a media star on Radio 2UE and Channel 9's *The Midday Show* and as a writer of entertaining and insightful newspaper and magazine columns.

Here's a sample of his literary style. In *Rugby League Week* in 1994, though hurting badly with his depression and addiction, he was still capable of penning this piece on the art of sledging:

> Sledging comes in many varieties. If you stand out in any way then you're a candidate. For example, if you're getting on, it's the old grandpa or has-been line. If you're overweight, it's the old fatso line. If you're skinny, it's the old refugee line. And race and skin colour always draws extra comment. Like every player, I copped my fair share of sledging. While it generally didn't bother me, I must admit one line hit home. When I was starting out at Souths in Brisbane, the then-coach of Norths, Barry Muir, decided he was going to intimidate me. Like most 19-year-olds, I had a few pimples. Muir homed in on this and started calling me the 'Zit-Zit Man'. Parramatta's Steve Ella was the 'Zip-Zip Man' and I became the 'Zit-Zit Man'. I can laugh about it now, but I took it to heart at the time . . . Stuff like 'Jackson, I've seen better centres in a chocolate' I can handle . . . I remember playing for Brisbane at Penrith one day. It was a packed crowd and everyone was still and silent as the hometown hero Brandy Alexander lined up a kick at goal. Our big prop Sammy Backo had just come back from injury and was carrying a bit of weight. He was standing

> behind the goal-line and it was dead-quiet. Then this bloke yelled out: 'Hey, Backo! You've got an arse that would do Dumbo proud!' Of the 13 Broncos, only Sammy didn't laugh. I can't have a spray about sledging without mentioning my old mate Craig Coleman. Tugger is a champion sledger. He talks at 5000 miles an hour for a start. That means he can fit about five minutes worth of talk into 30 seconds. One day against Souths at Seiffert Oval I kicked the ball out on the full three times in a row. Tugger's response was: 'F–king Jackson, he can land the ball on a 20 cent piece. Pity it's in the pocket of a bloke in the grandstand!'

To his friends, Peter Jackson seemed to have it all. He had a beautiful wife in Siobhan, three gorgeous kids – Lucy, Jim and Ned – a dream home near the beach at Stanwell Park, south of Sydney. But away from the laughs and the limelight he was fighting a desperate losing battle against his demons. He spent long periods struck down with depression and blinding headaches. At some stage he became dependent on heroin. He checked into a rehab clinic for five weeks, but neither that nor the promise of his career nor the love of his family could prevent his final spiral. His wasted body was found in a motel room after a suspected drug overdose. Peter's death was a terrible shock for all who knew and loved him. We knew he'd been ill with headaches, and all his old team-mates, like me and Ricky Stuart and Wayne Bennett, too, kept in touch by phone. Typically Jacko, he asked us not to send him flowers – 'Just money and beer for when I'm better!' Peter and Siobhan were the kind of friends to Kim and me that, even if you didn't chat on the phone every week, you knew they were close. Kim was very attached to their daughter Lucy.

Kim, as ill as she was herself with cancer late in 1997, travelled south with me to join 600 other mourners for a beach service at Stanwell Park and to farewell our lost friend and pray for him as his ashes were scattered over the waves. Gary Belcher gave a moving tribute there on the sands, and recalled how Jacko loved a party. 'I couldn't keep up with you, Action, so I gave up long ago,' Gary said. 'Mal could, Eddie Muller could, Cement and Kevvie could, Mick McLean and, of course, Siobhan as well. Laurie Daley in his younger days got top marks in his "Jacko's party hard and play even harder" apprenticeship. Des Byrne tried to keep up, but you had youth on your side back then, mate. So what happened? How could it get so bad? For someone with so many friends, who was loved by nearly everyone he met, why couldn't we help? I know it's too late now, but I wish I could have said goodbye. I wish we could just play one more game together, you throwing long balls, Mal running into space, me there to finish off your great work. The hugs at the end, a few beers, some belly laughs and then goodbye! I love you, Jacko. It'll never be the same without you.'

It was just a beautiful, beautiful funeral. Mick McLean and I took Peter's ashes out into the waves in a rubber ducky and they were scattered over the water.

'Better Man' by Pearl Jam was played for Siobhan. I started crying. It was a celebration of Peter's life, rather than anything too sad. As it came to a close, Kim and I said a prayer for Peter and made our way up the beach. As we walked hand in hand, Kim sick and suffering from her chemotherapy, I could not help wondering if the next funeral that many of us there would attend would be hers. How tough must it have been for Kim?

But long before all that, back in 1987 when Jacko and Badge Belcher and Mal and I were so much younger and making our way at Canberra, Wayne Bennett, the brilliant tactician and iron-hard disciplinarian, was a revelation. None of us kids had ever experienced anyone like him. He couldn't give a stuff about being popular and making pals as he knocked us into shape. One day, Canberra's then chief executive John McIntyre was chairing a meeting at the Leagues Club of all three grades: the firsts, reserves and Under-23s. At one point he introduced a young bloke who was overweight, the size of a house, and declared: 'Gentlemen, this young man wants to play for the Raiders. Wayne, what can you do with him?' Wayne looked at the young fellow and said with extra ice in that intimidating drawl of his: 'John, I'm a coach, not a miracle-worker!' The poor young bloke's face just hit the floor. Then Wayne said, 'Get 'im outta here!' The whole room went deadly silent. He has never been afraid of saying what he believes has to be said, and if someone's feelings are hurt, then that's how it has to be.

My first full game in the top grade was in Round 8 of 1987, when we beat North Sydney 46–11. I made 19 appearances in first grade in 1987 under Wayne, including an appearance from the bench in the grand final. Laurie Daley, giving his first impression of the new kid from Ipswich, said: 'We made our debuts together at Canberra in the halves in 1987, and I remember thinking, "Who is this chubby, overweight kid?" Kevin's form that year was outstanding and he must have been close to Origin selection. I felt sorry for him because he had to make way for Mal Meninga, who came back into the side for the finals after recovering from a broken arm. Kevin was on the bench for the grand final against Manly, and made an appearance towards the end of the match, but he can consider himself unlucky not to have been in the starting line-up.'

We played Manly at the Sydney Cricket Ground in a 31-degree heatwave. It was the last grand final ever played at the SCG and the Raiders thought there could be no better occasion to win our first grand final at our very first attempt. But by the time I came on, in the 52nd minute, to replace Mal Meninga, the game was pretty much out of our reach. Kevin Ward, a big Pommy prop who had just got off the plane from the north of England, was a powerhouse and despite the stifling conditions he beat up our pack. Cliff Lyons's quicksilver magic did the rest. They downed us, 18–8.

Losing was a bitter, but probably necessary, experience for us. It's the accepted wisdom that before you win a grand final you have to lose one, and our loss taught us plenty. We came into the match on an emotional high. We were the sentimental favourites, not just with our own fans but with every other team's as well. The pre-match build-up was overwhelming and, as so many other teams have before and after us, we may have lost intensity the moment we qualified for the premiership decider. Wayne and Don did their best to keep us focused, but Mal, Badge and Sammy Backo, who'd been on a semi-final rampage, were quiet on the day. Only Jacko played to his potential, recovering, after Ron Gibbs did his impersonation of a guided missile and buried him in the SCG turf, to be our best back.

We all launched ourselves into season 1988 determined to go one better and win the comp that year. I was determined to hold down a regular spot in the firsts, but it was not to be. If I had any misconceptions that playing first grade was a walkover, I learned my error soon enough. There were some excellent inside backs such as Ricky Stuart, O'Sullivan and Ivan Henjak (we were called the Mosquito Squadron) on the Raiders' books, and I have to confess that my commitment then may not have been what it is now. At the end of 1987, Wayne left Canberra to return to Queensland to coach the new Broncos team that came into the comp in 1988, and his replacement at the Raiders was Tim Sheens.

Tim and I got off to a bad start. I make a point of never being late for anything, but for some reason I fronted 10 minutes late for one of his first training sessions. He didn't take kindly to it, and I never felt he had confidence in me after that. I played just nine matches for the Raiders' top grade in 1988 and, in spite of being picked for the Queensland State of Origin squad, only seven in 1989. Canberra was a learning experience. Even though we lost the grand final in 1987, I was in the thick of things all through the lead-up week, and being on the field in the big game, if only for a few minutes, was the highlight of my career up until then. Even though I preferred to play five-eighth, in my Canberra years I proved myself as a utility player who could be used at centre, half and lock as well. As a lesson in *life*, my time in Canberra was also valuable. I had never really been away from home before and it made me grow up.

My options were wide open for season 1990. Canberra had made me an offer to sign on again, but I was disenchanted at not playing enough first grade. I don't believe I figured in Tim Sheens's plans. He obviously thought there were other players in the club better suited to first grade than me, and not picking me was his right as coach. But I was, after all, 22 and it was time to establish myself. St George had approached Steve and me to play for them. But deep down I wanted to play for the Broncos. Even though I didn't want to leave Steve, who had decided to remain a Raider, in Canberra, I was keen to return home, to play with Kerrod who had become the Bronco, Queensland and Test hooker. I wanted to be close to my family again, to hook up once more with Wayne Bennett, whom I admired as a man and a coach. And, most of all, I wanted to marry Kim and start a family.

But there was one big problem. Much as I wanted to be a Bronco, they were not exactly tripping over themselves to get me on their books. After all, they already had a handy five-eighth by the name of Wally Lewis. But nothing ventured nothing gained, and I rang Wayne and was straight with him. 'What are my chances at Brisbane?' Understandably, perhaps, Wayne didn't sound too positive about it all, so I gave up hope. Then, just as I was about to re-sign with the Raiders, I got a phone call from Wayne. 'Kevvie, I've found a vacancy for you here,' he said. There was not a lot of money involved. In fact, Brisbane offered me less than I was getting at Canberra. But I talked to Kim and we didn't hesitate. We packed our bags and headed north to Brisbane. I thought I'd get a fair go there.

CHAPTER THREE

# A HOT RECEPTION

I was just 11 years old when Wally Lewis first burst into the sporting headlines. He was this young kid with long hair playing his first match for Brisbane Valleys and he scored three tries. From then on, as he starred for Valleys, the Broncos, Queensland and Australia, he was a hero to me. Wally is, simply, the greatest player I have ever seen, and when I arrived at Brisbane from the Raiders in 1990, as a young five-eighth yet to establish himself even as a regular first grader, he had a mortgage on the club's No. 6 jersey. I had no illusions when I became a Bronco. I reckoned when I joined that the best I could hope for was to get a few games at five-eighth when Wally was on rep duty, maybe play centre when he wasn't, and hang in there until Wally, who was then 30, retired. Then I would succeed him as the Broncos' regular five-eighth. If I'd done all that I'd have been more than happy. I never dreamed that in my first season at Brisbane I would be the only Bronco to play every first grade game, *and at five-eighth.* That I would also make the Queensland State of Origin squad, be named the Dally M Players' Player of the Year and the *Courier-Mail* Queensland Rugby League Writers' Player of the Year, win the Broncos' own Best and Fairest poll and be selected for the Kangaroo tour of England and France. If someone had told me when I was playing my first games for my new club that all that would happen to me in 1990, I'd have told them to go book into a head clinic.

Just before Kim and I arrived in Brisbane to move into a house we were renting from Alf Langer, Broncos coach Wayne Bennett shocked the world of league when he sacked Wally as skipper and replaced him with his great friend, the Broncos and Australian centre Gene Miles. At the start of the season Wally was injured and I played in his five-eighth spot. I assumed I was just keeping the King's throne warm until he returned from injury. I started the season strongly, and immediately rekindled my teenage Ipswich combination with halfback Alf and twin Kerrod. But it was still another bombshell when, on Wally's return to fitness, Wayne kept me at five-eighth and moved Wally to lock. All this was a mighty kick in the guts to the proud Lewis. But although I copped it from Wally's legion of fans, who blamed me for their idol's misfortune, the man himself certainly never took his frustrations out on me. If he did resent me, he hid it brilliantly. Wally was generous to me. He offered me advice and was always friendly. I got a huge amount of confidence from that and it helped ease the pressure

I was feeling. I was just happy that Wally was playing with me and not against me.

Here's how Wally today recalls the situation: 'I hadn't seen Kevvie play much, but I knew he had some talent. Everyone knew a great deal about his brothers Steve and Kerrod, but I reckon Kevin suffered from an identity crisis. Wayne Bennett knew Kevin could play the game, otherwise he wouldn't have received an invitation to join the Broncos. I never had a problem with Kevin, but with Wayne Bennett. I knew my exit had been planned by Bennett, and even if Kevin had 47 shockers it would have made no difference. I'd known of Bennett's fierce admiration for Kevin for a couple of years, so once he came to the club the writing was on the wall. Kevin came into a situation of uncertainty and the bad water had yet to settle. During the season, he came up to me and said: "Wally, if I knew this shit was going to happen, I wouldn't have come here." I respected him for saying that. I told Kevin it had nothing to do with him . . . he was doing all that was asked of him by playing good football. I remember at the presentation night that year the club never gave me any recognition for my years of service. They didn't even mention my name, and I was dirty about that. I went and stood in a corner to have a drink, then Kevin and Allan Langer came up to me. Kevin pulled me aside and apologised for the way things had turned out. I told him to stop apologising because he had nothing to be sorry about. He is one of the few blokes at the club I regularly keep in contact with.'

As glad as I was to get my break at the Broncos in

1990 – and there was no way I wasn't going to make the most of it – I felt for Wally. He'd had a horrendous year. As he told *Rugby League Week*'s Tony Durkin, 'When the clock strikes midnight on New Year's Eve, I'll be the bloke cheering the loudest.' He'd be saying good riddance to a year to forget. How's this for starters? He was caught with his family in the San Francisco earthquake, was sacked as Broncos skipper, lost his five-eighth spot to me, tore a hamstring, missed only his second State of Origin match in 11 seasons, came back for Origin II but was fined $5000 for swearing at a touch judge, broke his arm, was out injured for the Test against France in which he would have broken Clive Churchill's record for captaining his country in Tests, quit the Broncos for the Gold Coast, and was ruled medically unfit for the Kangaroo tour. It says a lot about Wally's supreme talent that today, long after his retirement, the disasters are largely forgotten and all we remember are his many magic moments in our game.

It was wonderful being back in Brisbane, close to Mum and Dad and my brothers and Kim's family. We fell into the old family get-togethers as if we'd never been away. We immediately struck up strong friendships with the Broncos players and their wives or girlfriends. Kim met Michael Hancock's partner Janey Dopson at a football presentation night and they became inseparable mates. 'I don't know why we were such soulmates,' Janey says today. 'Somehow we just clicked that night and talked for hours. We had a lot in common and never ever had a bad word between us. We came from similar families. We were both pretty laidback and enjoyed a good time, though she was a peacemaker and I'm a bit more fiery. We followed Kevin and Michael to England on the Kangaroo tour in 1990. We stayed about five weeks and then when it was time for us to come home I moved in with Kim for four weeks until the guys returned.'

Kim and Janey had the time of their lives when they were together. 'We used to like to go out and get on the drink,' laughs Janey. 'We were pretty good drinking partners. We'd go to the odd movie, but basically we'd go out to have a big night on the town. With each other, other girls or with the guys. One of the best times Kim and I had was when we went to my hometown, Stanthorpe, for the Apple and Grape Festival there a few years ago. We had a huge weekend. When she got sick, we'd often have a laugh about that weekend.'

Kim and I were renting a house from Alf at River Hills. He was a damned tough landlord and God help me if ever I was late with the rent. When we went away on the 10-week Kangaroo tour at the end of the season, he demanded that I give him 10 weeks' rent in advance. I handed over the money, but let him know I wasn't happy about it. Suddenly he had a big smile on his face. He was having me on!

Because Kim and I were so happy in our life away from footy, I had no trouble switching off from the drama and intrigue at the Broncos. Our blissful homelife and all the wonderful things we'd planned for the years to come allowed me to concentrate on playing good football. I was fitter than I had ever been before, mainly thanks to Wayne and Kelvin Giles, a British athletics coach who came to Brisbane after stints at the Australian Institute of Sport and the Canberra Raiders. He introduced weight training and brought a new intensity to conditioning. He was a hard man who, like Wayne, wasn't out to win a popularity contest. We called him 'Mad Dog'. A lot of guys found the in-your-face Kelvin too abrasive, but I never had any problems with him. Being fitter helped me to play well consistently week after week and I never missed a match through injury all year. This, and having the confidence that comes with being accepted by team-mates and coach, added up to a strong season, probably ranking with 1992, 1997 and 1998 as my best in the game.

My normal game – which hasn't changed all that much to this day – fell into place. I was the linkman in a team of brilliant stars. In Jacko, Gene Miles, Michael Hancock, Chris Johns, towering fullback Paul Hauff and Willie Carne, we had the best backs in the comp and my job was to give them the opportunities to do their magic. In the early years, until I got more experience, I let Wally, Kerrod and Alf make the plays; they in turn capitalising on the hard work of forwards Greg Dowling, Andrew Gee, Mark Hohn and Terry Matterson. They'd get me the ball with the roll-on, then I'd free my outside men.

As for Origin '90, Michael Hagan in the first match and Wally Lewis in the second and third kept me out of the Queensland run-on sides, but I was on the bench for all three games and got onto the field in the first and third.

When the semis rolled around the Broncos were many pundits' pick to win the premiership. I was on a high after a season of achievements. As usual, pride came before a fall. It was Brad Izzard who lowered the boom and turned my high into a career low. The sandy-haired Penrith five-eighth was a powerhouse. He was about as wide as he was tall. Brad was one of the hardest runners in the game and in the major preliminary semi he ran right over me. I'd played against him before and handled him just fine, but this day at the Sydney Football Stadium he was hot and I was cold. His busts, running straight at my left shoulder, led to tries and we went down 26–16. Brad scored twice and was man of the match. I reckon it was my below-par defence in that game that has branded me with a 'can't tackle' tag to this day. Ever since that day, opposition coaches have run their biggest men at me, notably in our two grand finals against St George in 1992 and 1993 when Tony Priddle and Scott Gourley targeted me. Without success, I have to say.

Returning to the 1990 season, all the next week before our minor semi-final against Manly I got square eyes studying the video of my shocker against Izzard and decided that my tackling technique was at fault. I worked on my defence at training, getting huge men such as Brett Plowman to charge at me. Then, to rebuild my shattered confidence, I replayed videos of games when my defence *was* up to scratch. Kim, at home, told me not to get obsessed about that one poor match in a season of success and soon I had put the nightmare behind me. Brad Izzard had run roughshod over opponents throughout his career. I was by no means the first bloke he'd steamrollered and I wasn't the last. But I vowed there was no way he'd do it to me again.

Today Brad recalls his demolition of me in that semi. He says: 'It wasn't in the game plan to single out Kevin, but I knew with my size I had some advantage over him. I didn't think Kevin had a defensive problem, and I just put it down to the fact that I had a good day and he had a bad one. It's not often during a game that you are one on one against your opposite number, but in this game twice I ran at Kevin and managed to get on top. His body language didn't suggest he was affected by his mistakes, but I suppose deep down he would have been bothered by it. By putting Kevin under pressure, it forced the Broncos to give him more support in defence, which provided us with an overlap out wide. Sometimes, you see a player crushed by playing poorly in a big match and not be able to come back. I suppose Kevin may have been thinking after the match, "Do I really want to do this anymore?" All players get negative thoughts if they don't perform well, so it was vital for Kevin to hit back hard and put the experience behind him and learn from it. Which he did. Kevin knew he'd made mistakes, but he rectified them and has proven to be a quality player for a number of years.'

On the principle that you climb back onto the horse that's thrown you, I couldn't wait to get another crack at Brad in the final or grand final, but it wasn't to be. After a hard-fought 12–4 win against the Sea

Eagles – in which I won a points victory over Manly five-eighth Cliff Lyons and combined with man of the match Kerrod to score our first try – we were blasted out of the comp, 32–4, by brother Steve and my old Canberra mates, who then beat Penrith in the grand final a week later.

I thought I'd done well enough in season 1990 – my impersonation of a turnstile against Brad Izzard apart – to be an outside chance for the Kangaroo team that was to be announced on grand final night. I badly wanted to be on that plane to England and France. Ever since our backyard matches at home in Ipswich, it had always been my dream to be a Kangaroo. The only thing better than me making the team would be if Kerrod made it too, and the only thing better than that would be an Australian jersey for Steve as well. As it turned out, the Walters family scored two out of three. When Kerrod's and my names were read out, I was overjoyed and emotional. Kim hugged me and cried and I was engulfed in the congratulations of loved ones and team-mates. It was a big, big night. But while Kerrod and I were over the moon, Steve was deep in despair. On the flight from Sydney back to Canberra with his victorious Raiders team-mates, coach Tim Sheens read out the names of the Canberra Kangaroos: Belcher, Daley, Lazarus, Meninga, Stuart. Steve had missed out this time – to his bitter rival Ben Elias – but my older brother's green and gold days would come. The very next year he became a Test regular and that, as I've said, made us the first trio of brothers ever to represent Australia.

All up, I played five matches on the Kangaroo tour, against Wakefield Trinity, Cumbria, Warrington, Halifax and Hull. No Tests. Ricky Stuart was five-eighth and Alf halfback in the First Test at Wembley, which we lost 19–12. Alf and Kerrod, who hooked in that game, were scapegoats for the defeat and lost their spots to Cliff Lyons (who played five-eighth, with Ricky moved to Alf's spot at halfback) and Elias for the remaining two Tests, which Australia won 14–9 and 14–0. If we Broncos felt discriminated against, we didn't show it and cheered on the Test players in that classic Old Trafford Second Test when, with the score 10–10 with minutes to go, Ricky intercepted to put Mal over for the winning try, and also in the Ashes decider at Leeds. I can't talk for Alf and Kerrod, but I was just happy to be there, a part of one of the best sides ever. As in my early days at Canberra, I wanted to soak up the experience of the senior players and I hoped that some of the class of Mal, Bob Lindner, Andrew Ettingshausen, Cliff Lyons, Steve Roach, Gary Belcher and Laurie Daley would rub off on me.

You might say, though, that I made up for any football disappointments with lots of fun off the field. We had a ball, getting to know (probably better than was good for us) the pubs and nightspots of Manchester, where the Roos were based for the English leg of the tour. Strangely enough, considering the bitter clashes we'd had in the Sydney premiership, the Broncos Kangaroos, Alf, Mick Hancock, Chris Johns, Dale Shearer, Kerrod and I, and the Penrith boys, Greg Alexander, Brad Fittler, John Cartwright and Mark

Geyer, got on like a house on fire. At first the two groups were stand-offish. The Panthers thought we were the big-heads from Brisbane and we thought they were full of themselves as well. Those early impressions were way off beam.

Kim spent a short time in Manchester while we were based there. She flew over because she was missing me. It's good to be able to tell you that Kim was *not* around when ten of us guys got our bums tattooed. We walked into the tattoo parlour drunk, dropped our daks, and got 'Roos '90' etched on our right cheek. We didn't spread the word around the whole team but soon there were whispers that we'd had the deed done. The guys soon figured out a quick and effective method to get their tattooed team-mates to reveal themselves. At training next day blokes would be racing around hitting you on the arse and if you squealed you were incriminated. Chris Johns woke up the morning after he was tattooed, took a look at his arse and couldn't believe he'd let himself become the Illustrated Man. In a mad panic he rang his wife. 'Listen darlin',' he said, 'last night we had a few drinks and, well, we all decided to go and get ourselves tattooed.' His wife went, 'Oooohhh!' and started bawling, started howling. Chris tried to calm her down by telling her that he'd been having her on. 'Oh, no, no. I'm only joking,' he lied. 'I haven't got a tattoo!' Then he jumped in the shower, got a scrubbing brush and tried to scrub the tattoo off. Not surprisingly, it didn't work. It took him about a week to bite the bullet and call his wife and admit: 'Look, darlin', I really *do* have a tatt.'

For the benefit of team-mates and Manchester locals, Alf and I dusted off our old Ipswich party trick of fake fights. After years of rehearsals, we had it down pat, bashing each other and wrestling. We were so convincing that when we'd turn on a blue in a pub or on the street bystanders would do one of two things: make themselves scarce or intervene. 'Leave that poor little bloke alone,' they'd threaten me as Alf, with only a little help from me, hurtled against walls, tumbled down stairs into gutters and collapsed with a clatter among garbage bins. He's amazing. I think Alf learned how to pretend he was copping a belting from his brother Kevin. It's a skill passed among the Langer family. He's so convincing when he hits the deck that you swear he's an ambulance case. Alf makes me look like Mike Tyson, which is a long, long way from the truth. Once, in Manchester, Alf and I were walking up a busy street and there was a pile of green bags stacked up to be collected by a garbage truck. Alf said to me: 'Kevvie, throw me into these garbage bags.' So we got stuck into a mock fight and I grabbed Alf and threw him into them. A couple of big Englishmen saw it all and rushed to Alf's aid. They pinned me to the wall and were about to start whacking me to pay me back good and proper for bashing up the little blond fellow lying unconscious on the ground. Alf opened his eyes long enough to see that I had bought myself some real trouble and after making me sweat as long as possible he leapt to his feet yelling: 'Don't hit him! It was all a joke!'

Call us big kids, but Alf and I still stage fake fights

and I can't see why we won't still be beating on each other when we're 60. It gives us a laugh, and there's a lot to be said for that.

It's a wonder Alf made it back to Australia in one piece. In Leeds one night we went out for a drink at a big bar after a match. Taxis were swarming around outside at closing time, picking up drinkers to drive them home. It was bedlam on the street. Alf decided he'd pretend the taxis were opposition players and ran out onto the road dodging the speeding cars. They were just missing him as he stood there until the last minute then sidestepped out of their way. He was so nonchalant. Passersby couldn't believe it. 'Look at this bloke!', they were saying as their mates joined them to witness Alf's performance. In front of the sizeable audience that had gathered by the roadside, Alf put on a real show. He walked backwards into the traffic, not even looking at the oncoming taxis. Then just as they were about to cream him, somehow he swerved out of their way. Only someone with his incredible reflexes could have pulled it off. Me being me, I said, 'Hey Alf, that looks easy!', and had a go. I got halfway across the road and suddenly all these cars were bearing down on me, *rrrmmm! rrrmmm! rrrmmm!*, so I did a big dive roll to safety and lay there at the side of the road shaking. And don't kid yourself the shaking had anything to do with the cold north-of-England night.

Another time on that 1990 tour, in France, we were in a little bar and had quite a few drinks and at closing time they threw us out into the freezing cold night. For reasons known only to himself, Alf decided to show his displeasure at the bar owner's lack of hospitality by taking off his pants, jacket and shirt and climbing up the outside of the building in just his underpants and singlet. By the time he made it halfway up, about 20 metres off the ground, a large group of people had gathered, so Alf started playing to the crowd and pretended that he was a suicide preparing to jump to his death. The bystanders screamed: '*Non! Non!*' One Frenchman actually moved his car, not wanting Alf to land on it. But I called Alf's bluff and yelled: 'Go on, you weak bastard . . . jump then!' Just when Alf was deciding whether to jump or climb ignominiously down from his perch, a resident watching the action from a balcony higher up tossed a bucket of icy water over him. That dampened his spirit as well as him. 'I've had enough,' he cried, as icicles formed on his drenched underwear. 'I'm out of here!' And he clambered to the ground.

I think it was that night, but it could have been another, when, with a skinful of booze on board, we screamed around the narrow cobbled backstreets of an ancient French town in the car of former St George forward Johnny Fifita, who was playing in France then. Don't ask me what happened, because I can't remember.

All good harmless fun. But in Perpignan things got nasty. I was out drinking with my Kangaroo team-mate John Cartwright and afterwards we were hungry and set out to find something to eat. We walked two or three kilometres from our hotel to the town where, because it was very late, most of the cafes, bars and restaurants were closed. Our hopes of finding a delicious crispy pizza were fading when we saw a pizzeria. Its doors were closed but the lights were on inside. 'Let's give it a go,' I said to John. We knocked on the door, hoping the owner would let us in and serve us a meal. The security window opened and the owner looked us up and down. He couldn't have been too impressed by what he saw, because he said: 'No, no, not open tonight!' And he slammed the window shut. We yelled, 'Come on, come on!', and banged on the door, much harder than before. He refused to answer. So we bashed, bashed, bashed again. 'Come on, mate! We want to have something to eat. Food! Food!' This time he did return, but not to let us in. He threw open the security window, holding a thing that looked like a small fire extinguisher. We laughed at him. 'Oh yeah, mate. And just what are you going to do with that?'

He showed us. He carefully aimed the cylinder of mace, which he kept handy to discourage menaces like us, and sprayed us all over. The pain! Our eyes were on fire. Scared and in agony, we ran around the corner and hid beside a car while some very heavy blokes from the pizzeria looked to find us and inflict more damage on us. Just then a police car pulled up and I said: 'Oh, thank the Lord! The cops are here!' But the gendarmes grabbed us and frisked us and said: 'Money, money – give us your money!' So we gave them what money we had on us, about 20 or 30 bucks, and they took it and said: 'Now piss off! And don't come back here causing trouble!'

The pain from the mace attack was excruciating.

For the next week we had to wear patches on our eyes. My face blistered and peeled as if I'd had a dose of severe sunburn.

By the time we touched down in Brisbane at the tour's end my wounds had pretty much healed and I could look back on a terrific experience. On that first Kangaroo tour I made I probably enjoyed myself a little bit more than I should have and I didn't play any Tests, but I have memories that will last a lifetime. I know I'll never be at a loss for stories to tell my sons and grandchildren in years to come.

I didn't have time to dwell on the tour too long, however, because we were almost immediately back into hard training for the Broncos' 1991 campaign. When we'd been knocked out by Canberra in 1990 we'd all vowed to go all the way the following year. And Kim and I had made a date of our own. After being engaged since 1988, we had decided at last to get married early in the new year.

CHAPTER FOUR

# ORIGIN ANGST

Kim and I were wed in Ipswich. It rained on our wedding day, which is supposed to mean happy days for the bride and groom and lots and lots of children. Kerrod was my best man, and Steve, Andrew and Brett were groomsmen. Siobhan and Peter Jackson both wrote poems which they read out at the reception. Jacko claimed that he wrote his one about me while having a few stubbies sitting on the toilet the night before. Whether he did or not, it was hilarious and had the whole joint in stitches. It read:

*There was a young boy from Ippie*
*Who on the football field was quite nippy.*
*He met a young glamour on the banks of the Bremer,*
*And went home covered in lippy!*

*It was obvious to all it was passion at first sight.*
*The stars in Unit's eyes and Kimmie's love bite.*

*She liked his cute bum and his little chip kick.*
*But what she liked most was his really big . . . ears.*

*Unit loved her blonde locks, her very good looks.*
*The way she walked, the way that she cooks.*
*But the thing big Unit loved most of all*
*Was the way she played with his left . . . toe.*

*Now the Walters clan bosses, KG and Sandy,*
*Knew that young Kevvie was a damn sight randy.*
*But no need to worry, as he dragged her to bed*
*Kimmie shouted, not till you shave off that second bloody head.*

*Their scene was Jett Park, Easy Street, all that stuff,*
*But for these two young lovebirds it wasn't enough.*
*They both thought there was much more to see.*
*So Kevvie and Kimmie – and another great player (guess who!) – headed off to the ACT.*

*It was cold, it was new, and a little bit lonely.*
*But they knew they were each other's one and only.*
*T'was the first time they shared a bathroom and bed,*
*So to make it a little easier they moved in with Boxhead.*

*Kevvie needed a spare room to park his 25th new car, so they had to buy a new place quick.*
*And to make sure they behaved, Buddy sent down young Mick.*
*Now things at the Raiders weren't working real fine,*
*And his contract at Canberra was almost out of time.*
*He needed to get cracking, he was nearly out of his teens.*
*So he gathered up his courage and headbutted Tim Sheens.*

*So they moved back to Queensland – yes, that was the thing.*
*Play for the Broncos and dethrone the King.*

*To Kim it was natural to play for Brisbane of course.*
*She always thought Kevvie was hung like a horse!*
*To make it at Lang Park, Kevvie had to work hard,*
*And once a month he mowed coach Wayne Bennett's yard.*

*The blood and sweat paid off, that's for sure,*
*'Cause in late November he was on the Kangaroo tour.*
*So de facto life was replaced by matrimonial bliss.*
*It started today in the church with a kiss.*
*It's the most important contract you'll sign in your life,*
*And tonight you can do the dirty as husband and wife.*

Wayne gave me a week off training and Kim and I went to Tweed Waters for our honeymoon. Billy was born nine months later. We had always planned to start our family straight away. Kim was just so keen to be a mother. In some ways she had been a mother-figure to her own much younger sister Kelly. And ever since she was a teenager she was always gaga over other people's kids. In Canberra and at the Broncos, she had always put up her hand when team-mates with children needed a babysitter. 'Just drop 'em off at our place,' she'd say when the parents wanted to go to dinner or a show. I wasn't real keen on having strange kids in the house, but Kim was crazy about it.

When Jack was born a happy-faced, porky little fella, the spitting image of his dad, Kim came into her own. She thrived on motherhood. She got a baby book where you stick in locks of your child's hair and record the baby's height and weight and the date when they first ate solid food and so on, and she updated the book all the time. She kept a baby book for Billy, too, but her cancer prevented her doing the same for Jett. She kept the little plastic bracelets the babies wear in hospital after their birth, and locked away in a box our sons' first teeth when they fell out. Kim was a loving mother, but could also be stern with the boys when she wanted to be. Pretty much the way she was with me!

When we became parents, Kim and I didn't go out as often. We loved staying home with the kids. Mostly I'd cook dinner. Kim hated the kitchen. She cooked a bit, mostly simple stuff. I'm a steak-and-three-veg bloke so it didn't matter that she was not a gourmet cook. We got by.

We moved into our home at Brookfield in 1997, just a year before Kim died. She loved it at Brooky and it was her pride and joy. We'd been keen on the house for a year or so, but it was too expensive for us, and then Super League came along and all of a sudden we could afford it. When we did go out, it was usually with footy friends after a Broncos game. As we got older, we didn't go to bars as much and started going to dinner at nice restaurants a lot more. We'd go to quieter places and have just a few drinks and listen to music in classy surroundings rather than go to some of the nightclubs we used to frequent where the sound system blew your ears out.

Kim was pals with all the Broncos wives, especially Janey Dopson and Sharon Gee. Kim and Janey spent lots of fun times together when Michael and I were off with the team. When we were in Brisbane, Kim, Janey, Michael and I would often do things as a foursome.

Janey recently described Kim and me in those days: 'Kim was quieter than Kevin, who was always witty and boisterous. They got on extremely well. They would have their little fights like we all do but they were very happy together and a good double act. Kim was always very supportive of Kevin when it came to football matters. I stick up for Michael, too, but when I saw how Kim supported Kevvie I was very impressed. She never worried about football groupies, and neither did I. We both had the attitude that we didn't want to have a jealous knot in our stomach, every time we went out, because other women were making eyes at our guys. Basically we thought that if the blokes were going to be unfaithful then that was their problem and their loss. Kim had her own life, too, and enjoyed a good time, but her No.1 priority was always Kevin and their sons. Kim was a fabulous wife and mother.'

Janey also recalled Kim's love for Jack, Billy and Jett. 'She could lose her patience some days and say, "These kids are driving me mad!" But she'd always wanted to be a mother. When Kevin was away she would load the kids into the car and take them to her father's house or to her mother's down the coast, or to our place. I'll never forget seeing her pulling up with her car filled with kids and bikes and balls. Nothing was a problem for Kim. She just got on with things . . . God, I miss her. It would be so good to still have her around and have her kick my bum and say, "Janey, come on! Get yourself *organised*!"'

Kim never loved the game of rugby league as I do, but she supported me all the way. She happily made the sacrifices all footballers' partners must. She came to see me play, whether it was for the Broncos or Queensland in Brisbane or Sydney or for Australia in the north of England. She had no worries about packing up our sons and taking them to England to watch me play on the 1994 Kangaroo tour, even though Jack was a toddler and Billy a baby. She was always happy for me when I had a good game. The night we won the 1992 and 1993 grand finals she beamed with pride. Many times I'd go to her if things weren't working out for me on the field and explain the problems I was having and nine times out of ten she'd come up with the right answer. She was a clear thinker and didn't overcomplicate things. In football, with huge contracts at stake and so much competition, players tend to take things very seriously, too seriously sometimes. But usually there is a simple solution to what seems to be the most unsolvable problem, and Kim had the knack of being able to cut through all the irrelevant stuff and zoom in to the heart of the matter.

She was a simple person and tried to keep everything in her life nice and simple. I'd often come home from training moaning and bitching and whinging about this and that and we'd have a talk into the night and, sure enough, next morning I'd feel like a different person. She was a maestro at calming me down and revving up my confidence. I used to get disappointed when I thought the Queensland State of Origin selectors weren't giving me a fair go. At times, I reckoned, I was dropped from the team unfairly. Once they sacked me the week after I'd won players' player of the match against the Blues. Kim would say: 'If that's the way they want to pick their team, well, it's their loss and not yours so don't worry about it.' And then I didn't.

She could also pull me into line. She was shocked when I got my bum tattooed when I was drunk and unruly in Manchester in 1990, but soon saw the lighter side of it. Then there was the time I came off second best when a playful punch-up with Broncos team-mate Peter Ryan and Chris Johns at the Paddington Tavern got out of hand and it made all the newspapers. Kim let me know I'd behaved like a goose . . . then told me to take boxing lessons from her dad.

In my early days I drank a lot more than I do now – most football players did – and sometimes I'd land myself in trouble. Kim would say: 'Well, there's no getting away from it, you've *really* been an idiot this time!' She enjoyed a drink, but in moderation. She helped me with my drinking in those wilder years. Footballers have earned a reputation as loud-mouthed, hard-boozing yobbos and occasionally I was guilty of that tag. When I did step over the line she'd grab me and say: 'Listen here, matey, you're drinking too much. You'd better quieten it down. Give it a rest for a couple of weeks.' I didn't always take her criticism that well, and I got cranky, but deep down I knew she was right and I did what she said. These days, I still enjoy a beer and good times with friends, but my over-the-top days on the drink are in the past. Anyway, heavy boozing has just about been stamped out of rugby league these days. There will always be notable exceptions, like those that have made headlines in 1999, but by and large the younger guys coming through nowadays don't drink nearly as much as me and my contemporaries when we were young and we all drank buckets of the stuff. The times have changed, and it's all about being professional. These days we have an intense swimming session at eight o'clock the morning after a match, so there's no more after-game piss-ups. And we train most days of the week, so if you show up at the pool hungover you can say goodbye to your career.

It was not alcohol, however, but complacency and sheer bad luck that destroyed the Broncos' dream of winning the comp in 1991. We started the season in good shape. We went undefeated through the Lotto Challenge pre-season comp, beating Penrith 20–16 in the final at the old NSW mining town of Broken Hill. At one stage we trailed 16–2. Then, as we've done so many times since, we went into top gear and overhauled the opposition. Our new forward signing, the pocket battleship Trevor Gillmeister, let us know how serious he was about making his presence felt at the Broncos when he whacked the fearsome Mark Geyer. MG and Gilly saw out the first half in the sin bin. Before Gilly came to our club, the word was out that the Broncos were soft in the forwards. After Gilly signed up, they didn't say that any more. Tough, hard and uncompromising, no-frills solid in attack and brutal in defence, Gilly set the mould for blokes like Alan Cann, Andrew Gee, Peter Ryan, Gorden Tallis and Shane

Webcke. Every team needs an enforcer upfront, and in these guys – the type where their opponents never quite know how far they will go to settle a disagreement on the field – we have had some of the best.

After the siren sounded at the end of that pre-season final, Alf, our stand-in skipper for the injured Gene Miles, hoisted the cup high. From that moment on, season 1991 was mostly forgettable. A string of losses, including defeats at Lang Park by Canberra, Balmain and Easts and a loss to Wests after Kerrod was sent off for punching Graeme Wynn, at one stage had us languishing in 11th place. Wayne was despondent and offered to stand down. Kerrod, Alf and I sat Wayne down whenever we could and persuaded him to stay on. He's not a man who gives much away in public, but believe me, no one is as emotional and passionate about the game as Wayne Bennett. Even though we rallied and won our last five premiership games, we had given the other semi-final contenders too much of a start and we missed the play-offs. We finished seventh, after winning 13 and losing nine.

One game was special, for two reasons. When I ran onto the field against the Gold Coast in the second round of the competition it was my 50th consecutive first grade game for the Broncos since I saddled up with them the year before. The other thing that made this match against the lowly Gold Coast a red letter day was that it was my first face-to-face encounter with Wally Lewis since he left our club at the end of 1990 to link with the Seagulls. All week before, the press was ripping in, trying to hype our meeting into a grudge match, and saying that Wally was going to turn it on to get even with Wayne. As often happens, the media's predictions of an all-in blue came to nothing and the game was played out uneventfully. We won, and at the end Wally and I shook hands after a spirited but good-natured tussle and said: 'Well played, mate.' It's also good to be able to report that, although there was tension between Wally and Wayne back at the end of his Broncos reign, today they have pretty much buried the hatchet.

While the Broncos struggled in the premiership, there was better news on the Origin front. Queensland won a classic series 2–1. It was spiced with close scores (6–4 to us, 14–12 to them, 14–12 to us) and violence. Origin has been packed with hairy moments, but few uglier than the mayhem of Origin II, 1991. It began when Mark Geyer, in a one-man war against us Cane Toads, appeared to chop down on my brother Steve, who had usurped Kerrod's Queensland hooking spot by then. Wally sprang to Steve's assistance and flew at MG. At halftime the pair sledged and chested each other on the sideline. Order was barely restored. I was just waiting for one of them to throw a punch. Fortunately neither did. But, gee, it looked as if they were going to, and I think they both wanted to, but sanity prevailed and they both held back. It would've been a good knuckle, actually, because MG's supposed to be able to throw 'em all right and Wally certainly can. After the break, Mark kept coming at us, and it was after his high shot on Paul Hauff that Jacko went berserk and set off after the much bigger MG. That's just mates sticking up for mates. It's all part of the game.

The 1991 series turned out to be Wally's last Origin hurrah. He skippered the team from five-eighth in each game, which meant the subs' bench for me. My nickname of 'Splinters' was beginning to hurt. I would have given anything to be out there on the field for that classic series. It had everything: huge hits, as Geyer, Blocker Roach, Paul Sironen, Andrew Gee and Martin Bella hurtled through the air at each other; some of the best tries you'll ever see courtesy of Meninga and Mark McGaw; miracle goals from the sideline; and more high drama than you'd see in a year at the Sydney Opera House.

I believe that my performances in the 1998 Origin series proved once and for all that I could compete at that level, but I'd be having myself on if I didn't admit that State of Origin has caused me a hundred headaches in my career. Although I've played for my state 23 times since my debut in 1989, nine of those appearances have been from the reserves bench. Apart from 1998 and 1999 when I was in the run-on side for all three matches, a combination of factors – patchy form, playing behind beaten forwards, erratic and to my mind inexplicable decisions by the Maroons selectors – meant I've never completely cemented my position in the Queensland team. As a proud Queenslander that's a blot on my career I could do without.

So many great games, so many wonderful players. There can be no standard of rugby league in the world higher than State of Origin. My first taste was as a kid with my brothers and the Langer kids in the terrace beside the Ron McAuliffe Stand at Lang Park, when we would sit entranced by the ferocity and skill on display. Our eyes were sticking out of our heads at the wild and wonderful deeds of those 1980s heroes – Wally, Artie, Mal, Chris Close, Johnny Lang, Rod Reddy, Fatty Vautin, Greg Dowling, and the blue baddies from south of the border, Steve Rogers, Tom Raudonikis, Eric Grothe, Peter Sterling, Les Boyd, Steve Mortimer, Craig Young. For weeks after those monumental clashes, we would act out all the big plays in our backyard games. Only I reckon our games were a bit dirtier. When I first played – for real – for the Cane Toads against the Cockroaches in Origin III in 1989 I was a green kid struggling to make my name at Canberra. Wally had a stranglehold on the No. 6 jumper, so I sat on the bench hoping for a call. I got on the field but that game was a dead rubber – we'd beaten the Blues 36–6 and 16–12 in the first two matches. In my debut game we won well again, 36–16, and Kerrod was man of the match. By the end of the 1980s, Wally had been joined by Kerrod, Alf, Gary Belcher, Michael Hancock, Dale Shearer, Marty Bella, Gene Miles, Peter Jackson and Trevor Gillmeister in the maroon jersey. At series' end in 1989, we'd won eight Origin games straight and taken two series in a row.

In 1990 I did better. I was named a reserve for all three games. Unfortunately, that year the tide was beginning to turn and a new generation of Cockies – Laurie Daley, Ricky Stuart, Blocker Roach, Ben Elias, Glenn Lazarus, Brad Fittler, David Gillespie – were paying us back for the beatings we gave the Blues in the 1980s. In 1990 we lost Origins I and II 8–0 and 12–6 and won III 14–10. The resurgent New South Wales spirit was personified by Ricky Stuart and Ben Elias. Ricky and Alf, and Ricky and I, have had some fun and games on the field over the years. Once, in an Origin match when Ricky's Blues had given us a beating, the siren went just as I tackled him. I was filthy on him because he'd played so well, and I had him on his back and was roughing him up. I snarled: 'I'd *love* to punch you in the face right now!' He looked up at me with a huge smile and said: 'Don't do it now . . . wait till I've finished my victory lap!'

Elias turned on a sequence of blinders against us in 1990 and was a bloody nuisance for years afterwards. When Benny packed down against Kerrod and Steve, especially Steve, for their club or State, the fur always flew. Benny was a brilliant and inspiring player, but as good as he was, he was even better at getting up opponents' noses. Benny would single out his opposite number and wage war. My brothers rose to the challenge. Plenty went on in those scrums as Benny and Kerrod, and then Steve, fought it out to establish themselves as the best hooker in league. In one Origin match, the game was just about over and we'd won and the selectors were meeting that night to pick an Australian side. Steve and Benny both wanted that green and gold jumper badly. As a scrum was about to pack, Steve said to Benny: 'Just take it easy in the scrum, mate. I've gotta play a Test next week!' You could see the steam coming out of Benny's ears. We always tried to belt Benny in Origin – just knock his block off – because he was such a competitor. He was a quality football player. You won't see one like him for a while.

Benny happily remembers his clashes with my brothers. Recently he said: 'I had nothing against Kerrod and Kevin and we got along well. With Steve, it wasn't exactly hate, but intense professional competitiveness. We had a number of heated battles over the years, but I loved playing against Steve because he made me raise the level of my performance. We wouldn't sledge, but took great delight in belting one another. We were competing for the hooking spot in the Test side, so naturally when it came to Origin we were fired up and sometimes emotions spilled over. Steve and I wouldn't socialise after a match, or we wouldn't until our mutual friends Laurie Daley and Ricky Stuart encouraged us to bury the hatchet. In our last Origin series in '94, Steve and I had a beer together and we have been friends since. There's no problem between us.'

There was, however, a problem between me and the Queensland selectors, and I spent Origin '91 as an interchange man again. That year, and throughout my Origin career, I sensed they lacked confidence in me. One big reason that I played my best Origin football in 1998 was that Wayne Bennett was Queensland coach and I know he believes in me. That made a difference. I knew Wayne would give me a fair chop. I was determined in 1998 to win the series and finally put to rest the age-old theory that I was no good at that level. Last year made up for a lot of hard years. But I admit that, in the seasons before, my feeling that the selectors had a vendetta against me affected my game. With the Broncos, which after all contains most of the Queensland Origin team, I have always felt in control. Some of my best games have been in grand finals. This is largely because I know I enjoy the trust and respect of Wayne and my Brisbane team-mates.

I know that often I've not played as well as I can for Queensland. We all have off-nights, and it is hard for backs to dominate when our forwards are copping a belting which, let's face it, was on the cards when we were up against Roach, Roberts, Sironen, Gillespie, Lazarus, Harragon and Clyde. Brad Fittler, who lined up against me for years, agrees: 'In the past, Queensland have blamed their five-eighths for their defeats, but in fairness to Kevin it's difficult to perform when our forwards have been on top. Queensland's forwards were able to give him a platform during the 1998 Origin series, and he was able to show his class.' Too many times, I reckon, Queensland coaches and selectors made me the scapegoat for losses, dropping me even after I'd been far from the worst player and even when I'd won best player awards. I always felt the selectors – and many in the media – wished I was Wally Lewis, and of course the great man's boots were big ones to fill (whoever takes over from Alf Langer at the Broncos and for Queensland now that he's given the game away will face the same problem).

I had been a Queensland reserve for a number of

years while Wally was still playing and then when Wally finally retired I came into the Maroons team. But I think I copped a bit of a backlash. They had me thinking I was the last resort. What with being dropped all the time, and negative reviews in the papers even when I thought I'd played OK, I ended up not believing in myself – and in a confidence game like rugby league that's fatal. When I was recalled to the Queensland team after being dropped, I'd try too hard, always feeling I was on trial, and when I try too hard I'm not at my best. I'd be out there on the field, thinking: 'Do I deserve to be wearing this jersey or don't I? Is there someone who's better than me who should be in my place?' In 1993 I was dropped for Origin III and replaced by Julian O'Neill. At halftime we were losing, and Julian got the hook – got pulled off – and I went on and laid on two tries and we won 24–12. I got pleasure out of that, but the bottom line is that I've underachieved for Queensland.

Wally Lewis has expressed some sound thoughts on my up-and-down Origin career: 'Kevin would be the first to admit he has been disappointing in a number of games, but I felt he was one of the players who really suffered because of our previous success. Everyone felt our success at Origin level would continue, but when we started to get consistently beaten Kevin was the one who bore the brunt of the criticism. It would have been a bitter pill for Kevin to swallow, but he has never been one to shy away from self-criticism.'

In my decade in the maroon jumper I've seen a lot of changes. When I started out in State of Origin, it was the days of blood and guts and bonding. Fierce camaraderie would be forged in the pub in the days leading up to a game, and by the time we got on the field we'd be happy to rip the Blues' heads off and eat 'em and we'd be glad to die for each other. That approach sure got results and made for some unforgettable matches, but, looking back, I have a few problems with the way things were in the 1980s and early 1990s. I think we made a bit too much of that 'great to be a Queenslander' thing. Sure, it worked sometimes. Once, Alf and I were out drinking until 5 a.m. while in Origin camp and we both put on a blinder in the game after having just one day to recover. So we thought, 'Hey, this is a bit of alright, Queenslanders can do anything', and went out on the drink again. Next game I had a shocker. It's hard to believe now that just because you're born north of the border you're somehow superior to someone who's been born south of the border. All that Cane Toad stuff got a bit out of hand, but now I think it's back to where it should be. These days, in Origin camp, we have a good time but remain focused on the game.

My brother Steve is another who never went for all the old hype. He said that the attempts to teach us to hate the guys in blue were a load of crap. He'd be in camp and some other Queensland player he might have known for a day would tell him how he'd have to go out and belt his Canberra team-mates and close friends like Laurie, Brad and Ricky just because they were from New South Wales. He'd think: 'Go and get stuffed!' And he's right. Hate may have worked for the guys in the old days, but I don't think players in today's game have that attitude. In our winning 1998 Origin series, under Wayne Bennett, we had fun but also spent more time talking about how State of Origin has evolved – how Queensland dominated at first, then New South Wales took command, and now there's a changing of the guard once more. New South Wales champions such as Laurie, Ricky, Brad and Lazzo are nearing the end of the road, while Queensland is back with a vengeance, thanks to young stars Gorden Tallis, Jason Smith, Darren Lockyer, Shane Webcke, Brad Thorn and Ben Ikin. The wheel is turning. Appreciating the history of State of Origin reinforced the point that we were part of rugby league history, and that was a terrific motivator.

There'll always be room for straight-out passion, however, and that's where Chris Close comes in. 'Choppy' is one of the old school, and images of him in the first Origin clash, jumper ripped from his back, throwing haymakers as a brawl raged around him, are vivid. Today he's the Queensland manager and, at Origin time, the old red mist descends. He got us together before the first match in 1998 and said: 'Listen, fellas, I'm not bullshitting, I've got a young bloke at home – he'll be watching tonight. Now,' he continued, his eyes shining, 'in years gone by the kid's had to go to school and put up with crap about Queensland losing, and I don't want him having to face all that again tomorrow because we lost tonight!' I immediately thought of Jack at his school, copping a bagging from his classmates, and I thought, there's no way I'm going to allow that to happen. The other blokes with kids all told me Chris's words had the same effect on them.

Back to 1991. At the end of the season an Australian side was selected to tour Papua New Guinea, and Steve and I were in it. Though it was a short tour, that PNG jaunt is a highlight of my career. We won both Tests: 58–2 in Goroka when I made my Test debut from the bench, and 40–6 in Port Moresby when I again got onto the field. When our plane landed in Port Moresby, more than 20,000 league-mad local fans were there to greet us. It was a sea of people come to see their green and gold footy heroes in the flesh. But, weirdly, these rugby league fanatics stood there in total silence, as if in awe of us. It was eerie – so many people and not a sound. I took a hand. 'This won't do!' I said. 'I'll get some noise out of them.' I stood at the top of the steps and waved my arms as if conducting a vast orchestra. The crowd took my cue and immediately broke into deafening cheers and whistles. 'Bella! Walters! Jackson!' they screamed. They knew all our names. What a welcome! Suddenly I knew how John, Paul, George and Ringo must have felt at the height of Beatlemania. In Lae, to commemorate our game there – and to mark a fortnight in which there had not been a single break-and-enter robbery – PNG prime minister Rabbie Namaliu declared a public holiday.

One of the highlights of that tour came at the end when the team hired two large fishing boats and filled them full of food and drink for a big day's outing. As soon as we set out we put on the music and started drinking. Somewhere off the PNG coast Peter Jackson said to me, Willie Carne and Chris Johns: 'I'm gonna jump overboard.' So, with the boat powering along at 30 knots, he climbed up to the top deck and leapt straight into the drink. What else could *we* do? I dived off next, then Willie and Johnsie. There were four of us bobbing around in the water. The captain turned the boat around and came back to pick us up. We clambered on board and the boat set off. A minute later, Jacko jumped overboard again. I followed, then the others. The captain, getting a little annoyed with us by now, did a U-ey and swung back to pick us up again. This time, though, as we were all treading water in the dark green ocean, he gave us some vital information. 'Boys,' he said, 'this water's shark-infested, and the next time you jump out of my boat I'm not coming back to get you. You can bloody well swim to the nearest land.' We looked around and there was no land in sight. We were in open sea. As soon as he heard the word 'shark', Jacko was running on water, scrambling over us, pushing our heads under the water, trying to get back on board and save his skin.

About lunchtime we put into an island. No one there – just us, a white sand beach to play cricket on, beautiful clear water for swimming, and lots of unusual fauna to photograph. At some stage of the fairly boozy proceedings I dozed off on the beach, my camera lying there beside me, and so I had no idea about what happened next. Anyway, when we returned home I couldn't wait to take the film out of my camera and give it to Kim to take to the chemist to process so she could share in the things we saw on our great day out. Next day she came home from shopping and she had the packet of snapshots. She'd obviously had a peek at them and she said: 'Oh, there's a couple of beauties in there which you'll want to put straight into our family album.' I said: 'You bet, that Papua New Guinea is a lovely place.' I began flicking through the photos. Kim was looking at me with this strange smile on her face. 'Now,' I explained as I held each photo up, 'that's where we went fishing . . . and those are volcanoes, and these . . .' I stopped dead when I came to the photo of my team-mates standing in a line on the beach with their swimming togs pulled down, exposing everything. I have my suspicions about who took the X-rated photo with my camera while I was passed out on the beach. You know how I know? All the guys were in the photo, except me, who was unconscious . . . and Jacko.

CHAPTER FIVE

# AS GOOD AS IT GETS

Wayne Bennett knew long before we took an unbeatable lead against St George in the grand final on 27 September that the 1992 premiership was ours. He said he knew that this year would not be a repeat of past years' disappointments the moment when we beat the 1991 premiers, Penrith, in a club game one icy August night at Penrith Stadium. 'Everything was against us,' he reflected later. 'The crowd, the travelling and playing on a Friday night . . . and the premiers were fired up for what was their last shot at winning a follow-up title. But despite those odds we won – and we won well. That night, I believe, we showed the qualities needed to win the premiership. All we had to do was finish it off.'

We did so, and how. After a loss to Wests, the Broncos breezed through the last seven premiership games undefeated to take out our maiden minor premiership. We whacked Illawarra and Saints in the semis and played St George again in the grand final.

Before the match at the Sydney Football Stadium, we felt very much the outsiders, even though we were hot favourites. When our trainer Kelvin Giles asked Saints ballboys and officials if he could borrow a couple of balls they had in a bag for our dressing room warm-up, he was rudely told no. And after the game, when we'd completed our victory lap, Kim and the other Broncos wives and partners were stopped from using the front gate to join us in the dressing room. Officials made them walk the long way around and run the gauntlet of abusive St George fans. Some say our grand final team that day was the strongest Broncos side ever fielded. The classy Julian O'Neill, at that stage a young star with the football world at his feet, was fullback. The three-quarters were Mick Hancock, Steve Renouf, Chris Johns and Willie Carne. Alf Langer and I were the halves and Terry Matterson was lock, with Trevor Gillmeister and Alan Cann in the second row. Kerrod was hooker. Gavin Allen and the colossus Glenn Lazarus were his props. The St George Dragons would be no pushover, with classy finishers like Mark Coyne, Ricky Walford and Mick Potter making the most of the offloads of towering forwards Tony Priddle, Scott Gourley and Dave Barnhill.

We led only 6–4 at halftime. Alf had scored a try

for us and Walford for Saints. But no Bronco was panicking. By tying up the ball for long periods we had been able to maintain enormous pressure on Saints' defence in the first 40 minutes without turning our ball-monopoly into points. Saints were scrambling desperately and we could see their huge defensive load was tiring them out. The dam hadn't broken at the break, but we felt it was only a matter of time.

We ran out after the break and struck almost immediately. Mick Potter ran a grubber kick out of his in-goal and set off upfield, but Willie Carne and I hit him hard and drove him into touch not far out from the Dragons' line. Seconds later, Alf jinked over from dummy half for his second try, carrying huge Tony Priddle with him. The joyous expression on Kerrod's face as he hurdled the prostrate Alf was priceless. Four minutes later, Gilly put Alan Cann into a gap and he beat five to crash over for our third try: 18–4 to us. But it was not the Broncos' way to protect a lead and we snapped into overdrive, hungry for more tries. Alf defied the wisdom that says ball security is paramount in your own quarter and right on our line he flung a 20-metre pass to Steve Renouf. Steve glided past his opposing centre, Rex Terp, and sped 98 metres to score in the 61st minute. Five minutes later, Alan Cann, who was known as a dour hit-it-up specialist and a bruising defensive forward, put on an astonishing, delicate, incisive sidestep that had Saints' Neil Tierney, who would have been expecting Alan to try to run over the top of him, grasping at air. Cann scored, then with a yell he slammed the ball down in delirious delight. I have had the photo of Alan's war-dance blown up and framed and it now resides in my lounge room. When he scored, there were still 12 minutes to go, but the celebration champagne was already tasting good. When the fulltime siren sounded, it was 28–8. In only our fifth season, we were the champions.

The unexpectedly large Queensland contingent in the crowd went wild, but down on the field, as we realised that we had hijacked the Winfield Cup, we were even wilder. We yelled, and laughed, and cried, and sang, and guzzled champagne and Powers beer. I grabbed Kim and we hugged. There in her arms at the Sydney Football Stadium I had never felt so wonderful. I basked in her love, in our win and in my own game. Everything I had tried in attack came off, and my defence was sound. My disastrous display against Brad Izzard seemed a long time ago. I told a reporter later that I had tried to put the nightmare out of my mind because I didn't want to dwell on the negative. 'But on days like today you can look back on things like that and say to yourself, "Well, that's dead and buried now. I can forget about it." That's what I'm saying. I probably missed one or two tackles today, but we won't mention those!'

But more important than my own performance was that we were the premiers. Feelings of happiness mixed with relief that the monkey was off our back at last. Our critics from down south had laughed at us and called us chokers under pressure. They said we

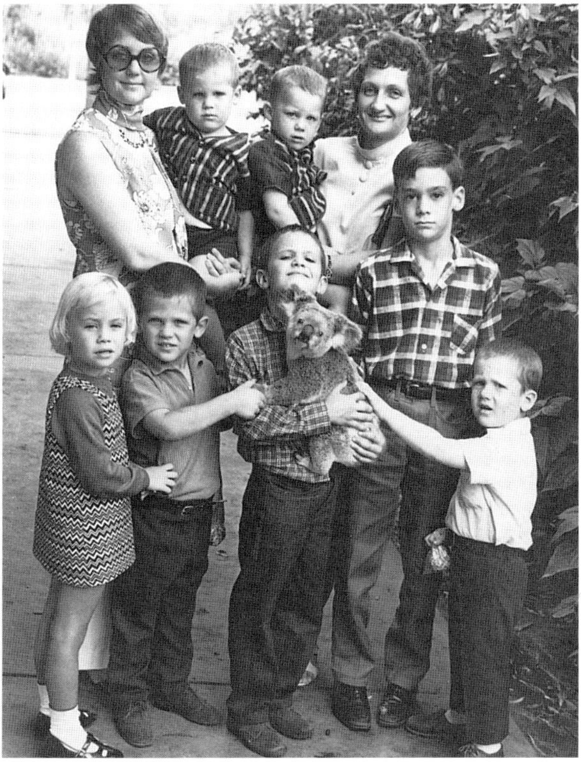

Some of the Walters clan at Brisbane's Lone Pine Koala Sanctuary. At the rear, left, my aunt Vivian is holding me and Mum is doing the honours for Kerrod. In the front row, from left, are cousin Caroline, my brothers Steve and Brett (with the koala), cousin Cameron and brother Drew.

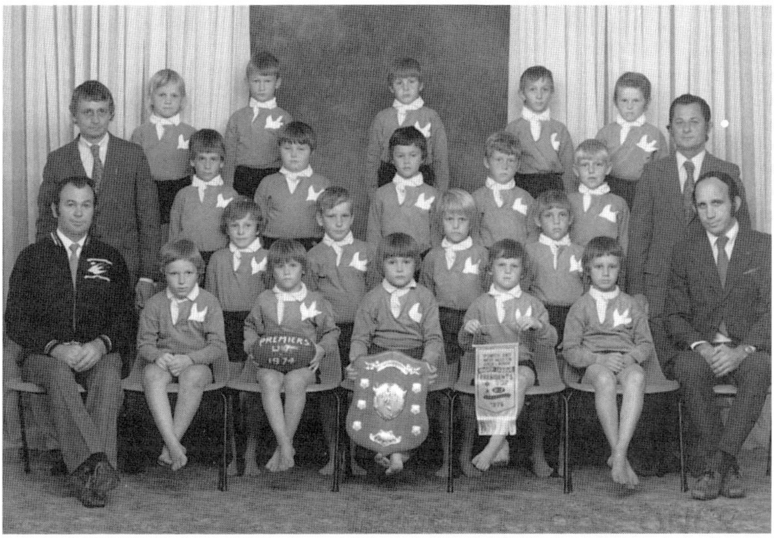


The mighty Booval Swifts' 1974 premiership-winning Under-7 team. That's me in the front row holding the footy, and Kerrod has the banner. Our dad KG is in the third row, far right.

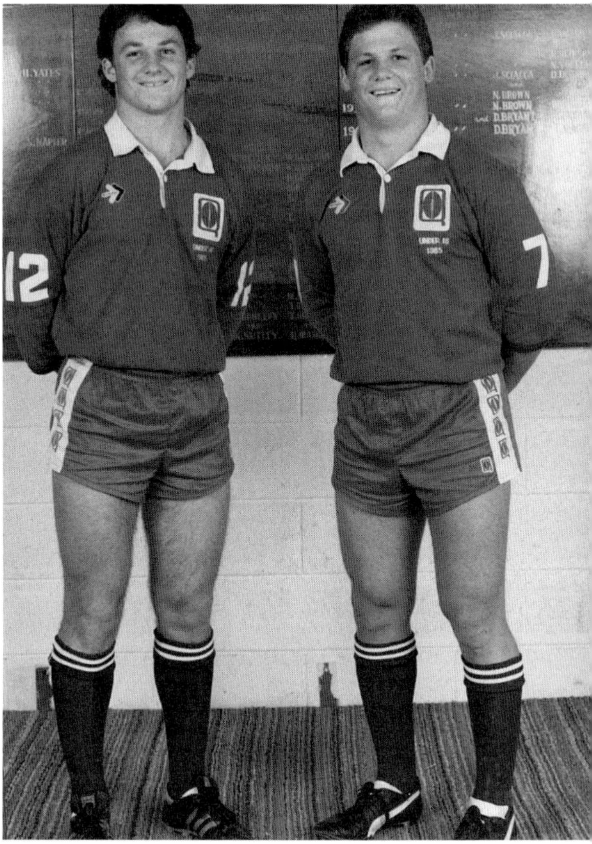

Kerrod and me, proud Queensland Under-18 reps in 1985.

Sandy and KG on the town. Mum and Dad were firm but loving when we were growing up and they encouraged us every step of the way.

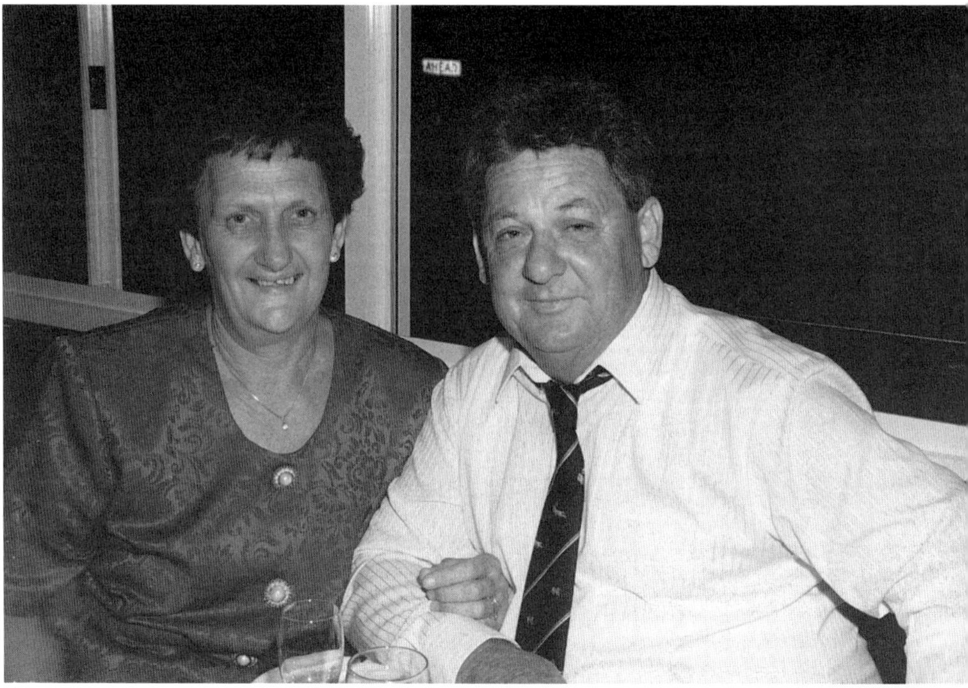

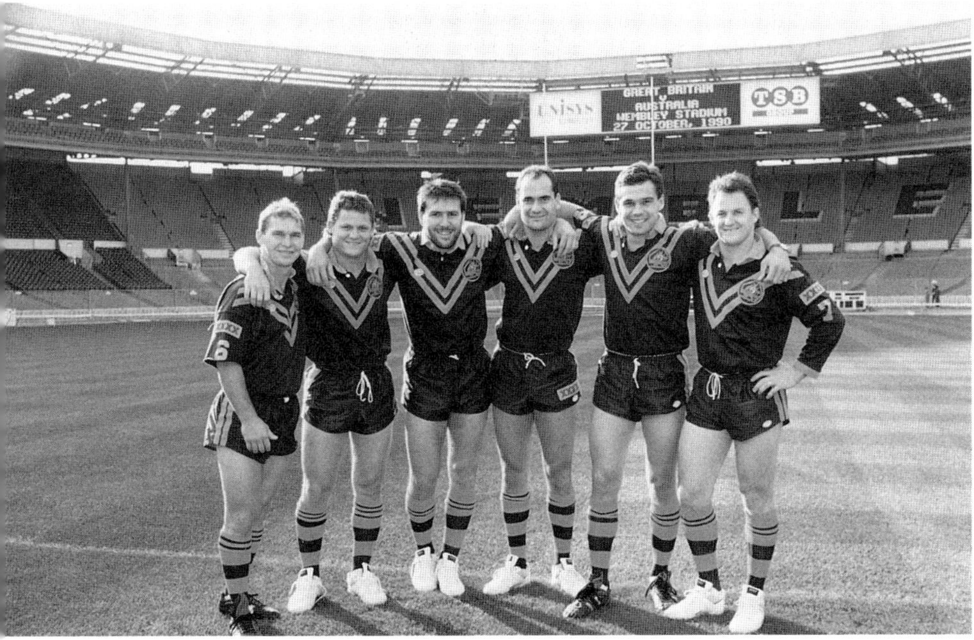


The Broncos invade Wembley. Allan Langer, me, Michael Hancock, Dale Shearer, Chris Johns and Kerrod, Brisbane's six 1990 Kangaroos, check out the hallowed London turf before the First Test in 1990.

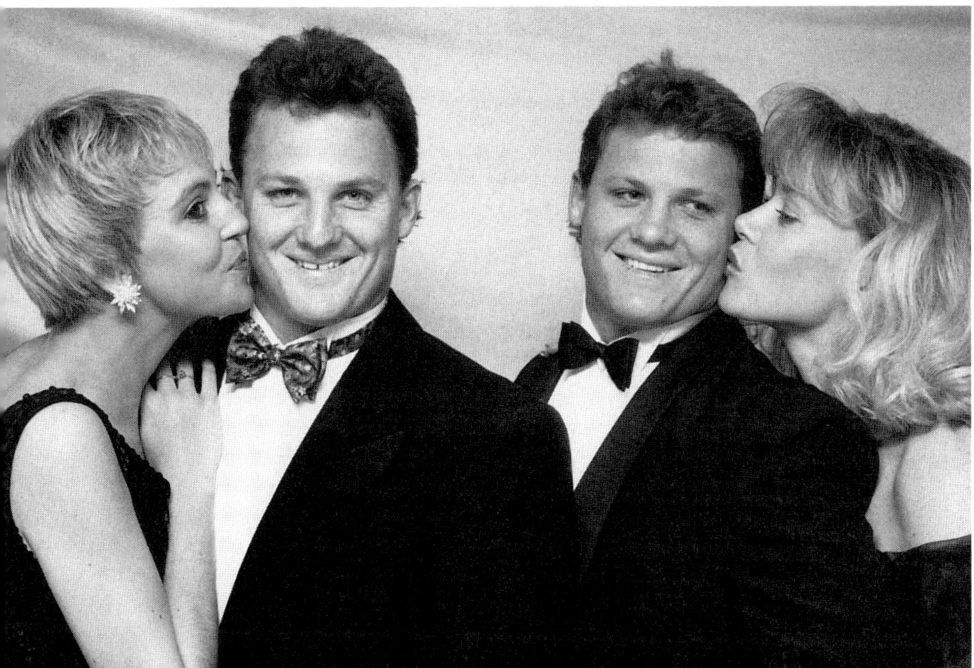

In 1990, Kerrod and I posed with our wives Maureen and Kim, both Ipswich girls. (Photo courtesy of Queensland Newspapers)

Kim, radiant on our wedding day in 1991, with her parents Lorraine and the great larrikin Buddy Facer.

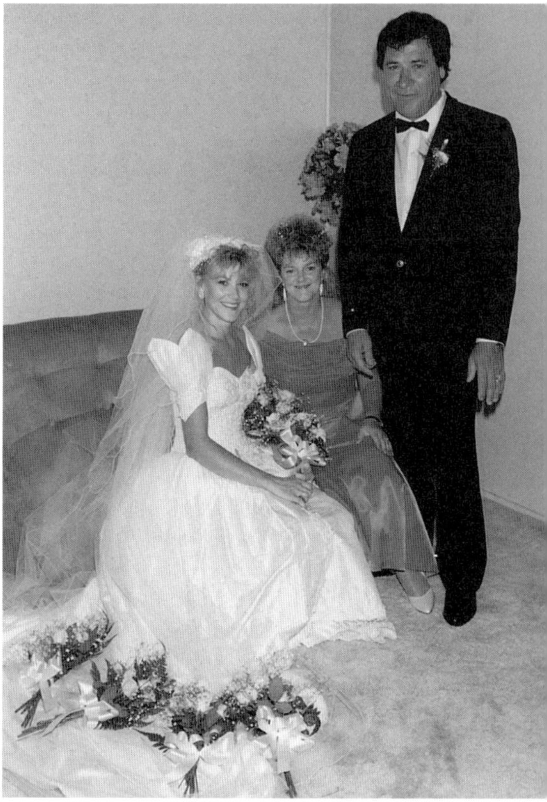

After the wedding we partied on at our reception at the International Motor Inn, Ipswich, and Peter Jackson recited his memorable poem. Before things got crazy we posed for the photographer. My brothers Brett, Andrew, Steve and Kerrod flank Kim and me on the left. The little boy is Kim's brother Kenny. Kim's sisters Kristy and Kelly are kneeling in the foreground and her sister Kerry stands second from the right.

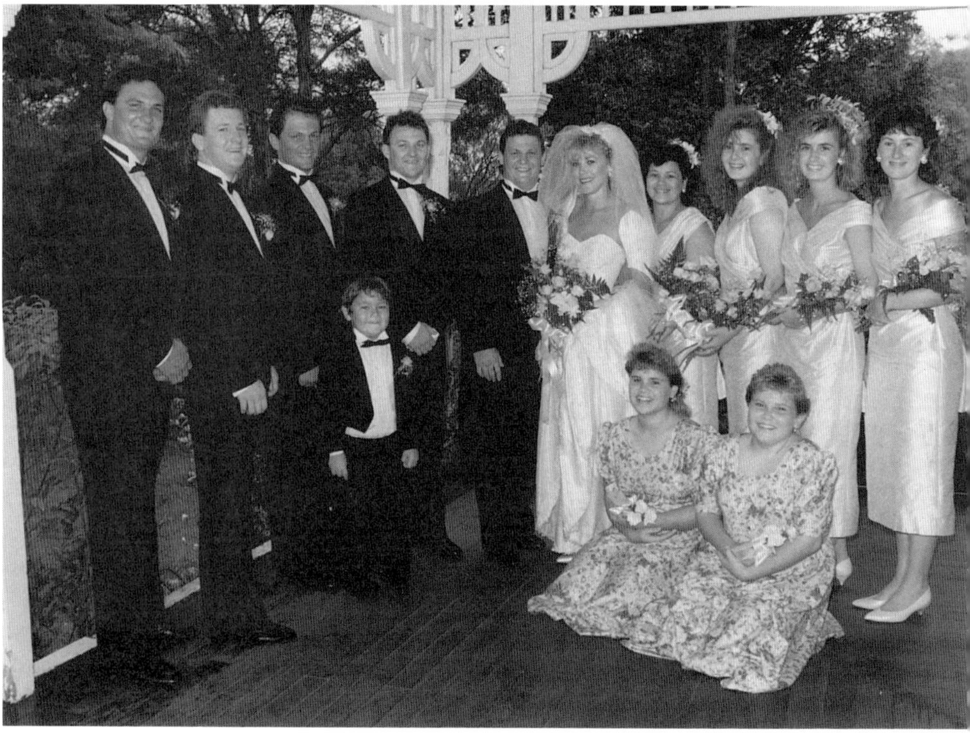

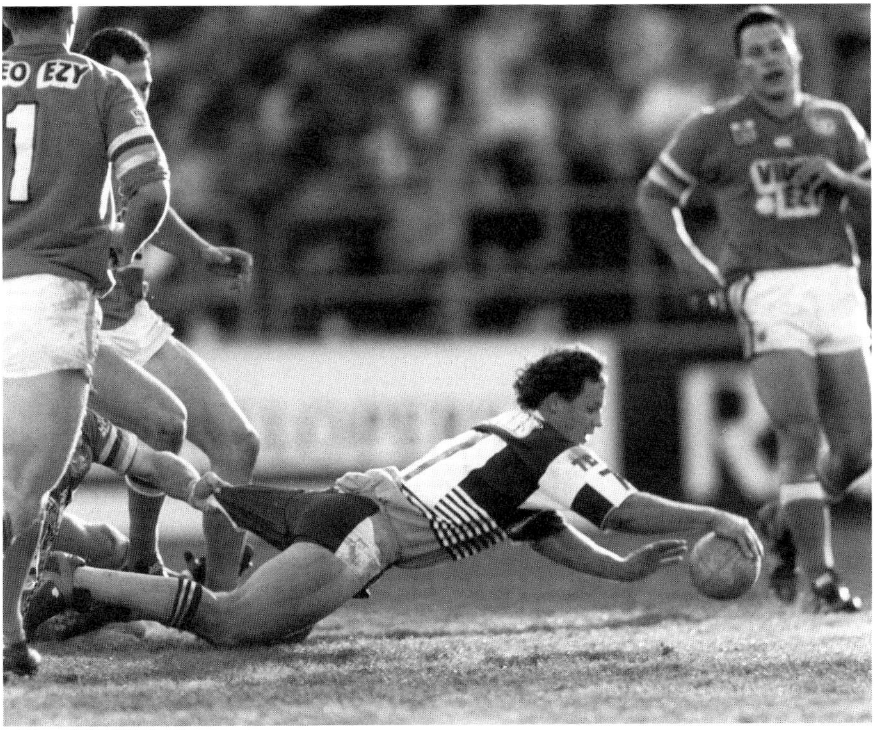

Sweet revenge as I score a try for the Broncos against my old team, the Canberra Raiders, in 1991. An unknown Raider tries to relieve me of my shorts. (Photo courtesy of Action Photographics)

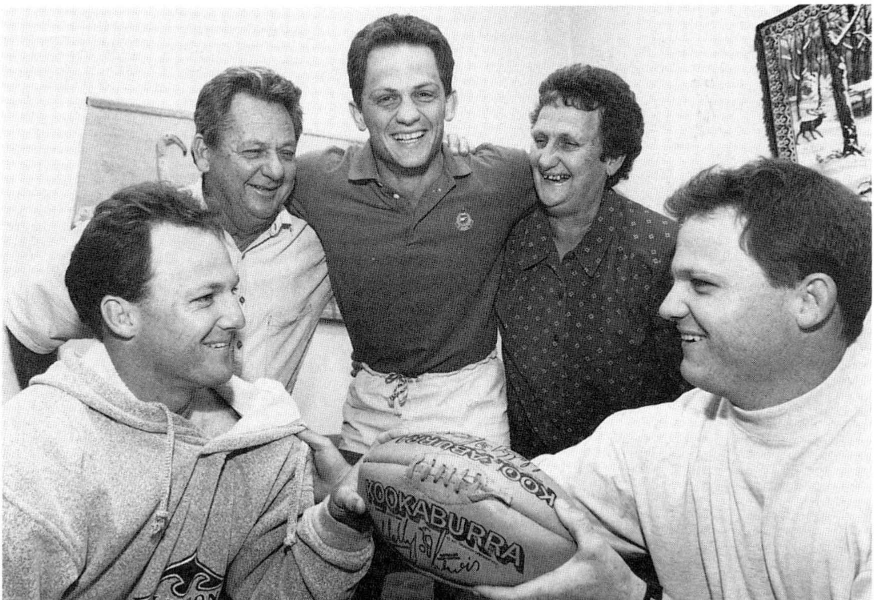


There were celebrations at Merton Street when Kerrod, Steve and I were all selected in the Australian World Cup team in 1992. Mum and Dad joined us at London's Wembley for the unforgettable final against Great Britain.

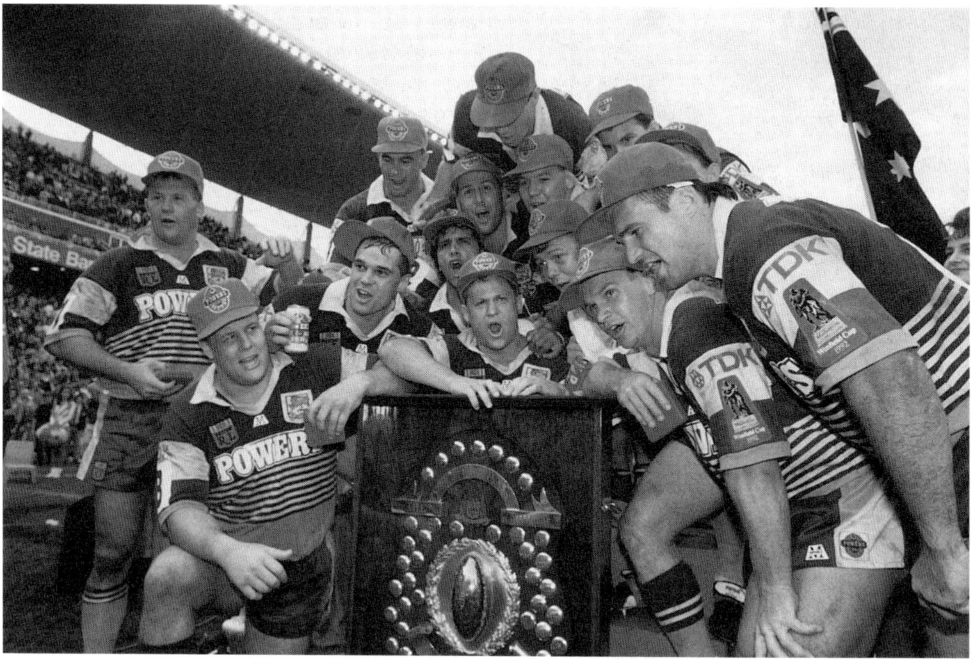


Premiers at last. After we beat St George in the '92 grand final at Sydney Football Stadium, Trevor Gillmeister, Glenn Lazarus, Chris Johns, Andrew Gee, Steve Renouf, Michael Hancock, Mark Hohn, Julian O'Neill, Peter Ryan, Alf Langer, Terry Matterson and yours truly ripped into the team song.

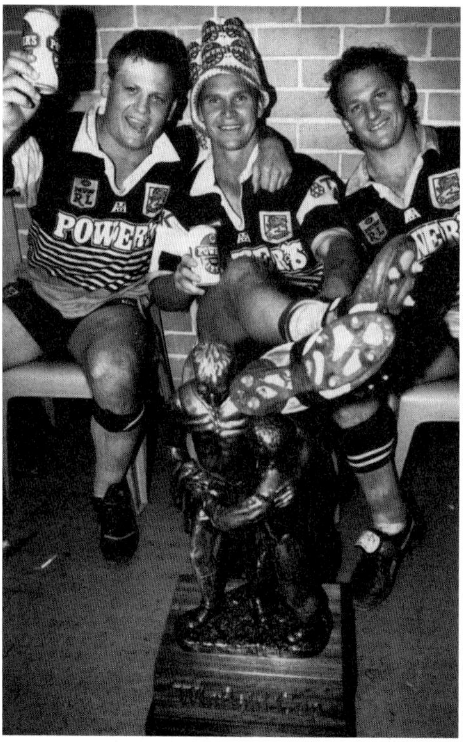

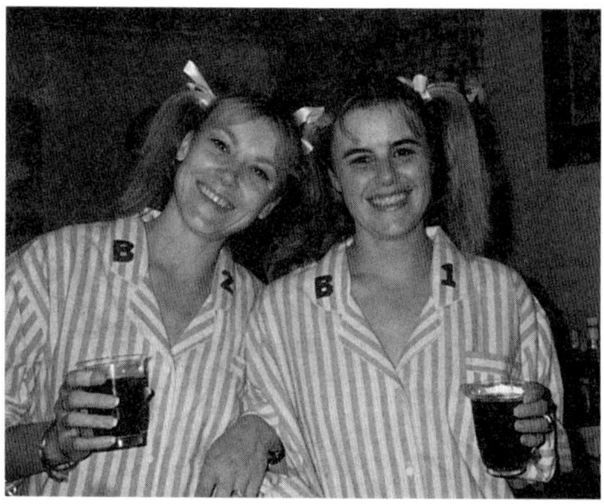

Bananas in Pyjamas. Kim and her great friend Janey Dopson as B2 and B1 at a pyjama party in 1993.

Allan Langer, sporting his infamous Powers beer hat, is a thorn between two roses: namely Kerrod and me, in the Sydney Football Stadium dressing rooms after the '92 grand final. (Photo courtesy of News Ltd)

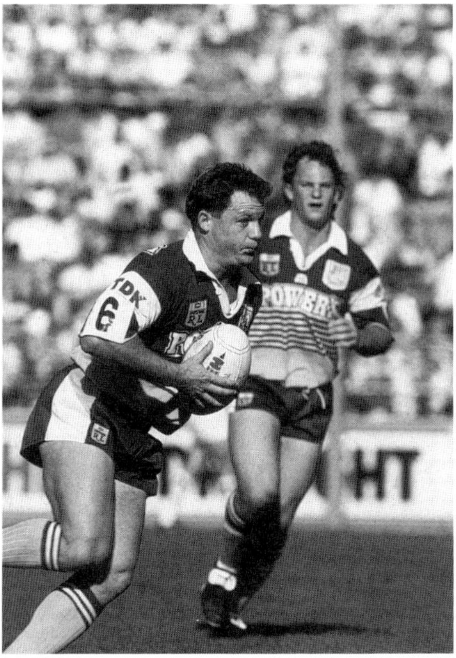

I weigh up my attacking options in the '93 grand final at the Sydney Football Stadium, again against Saints, with Kerrod in support. (Photo courtesy of *Rugby League Week*)

The Queensland 1994 Origin side lines up at the Melbourne Cricket Ground. We must have been expecting trouble from the Blues, because that's world boxing champ Jeff Fenech third from the left in the front row. Other faces in the crowd are the great Mal Meninga (sixth from left, back row) and Wally Lewis (centre, back row), and inspirational Chris Close (back row, fifth from the right).

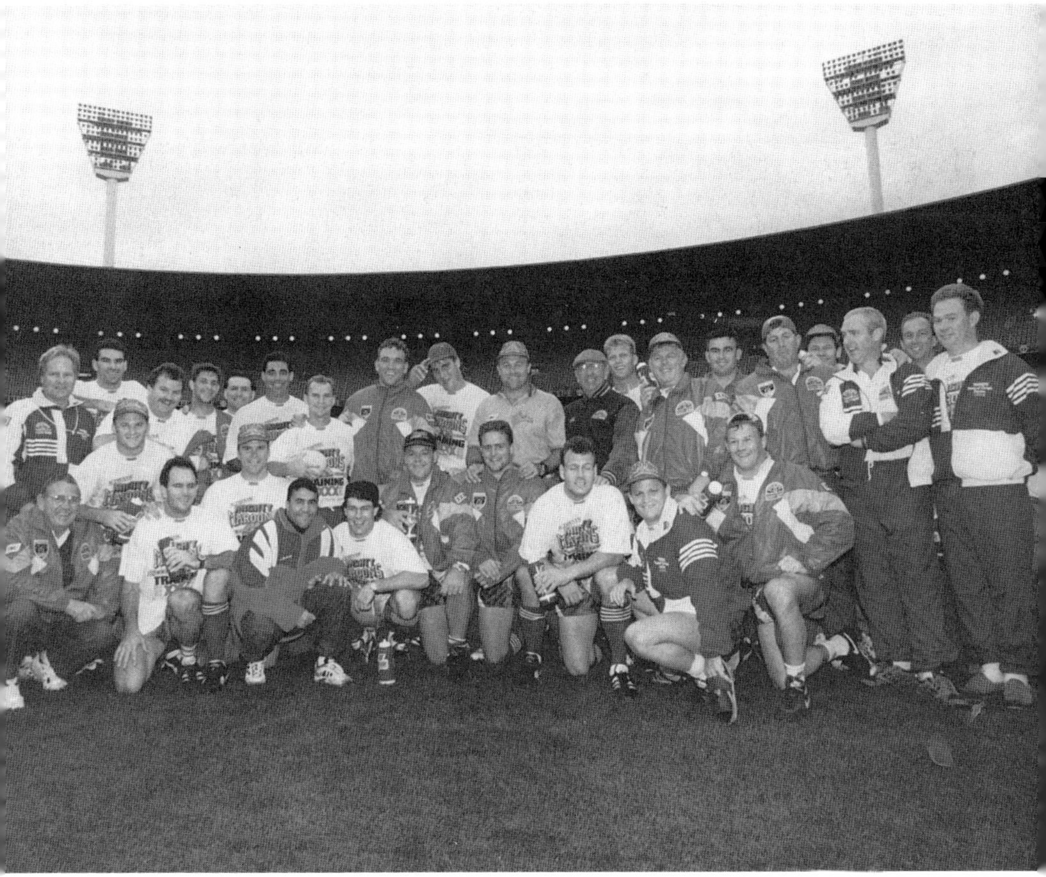

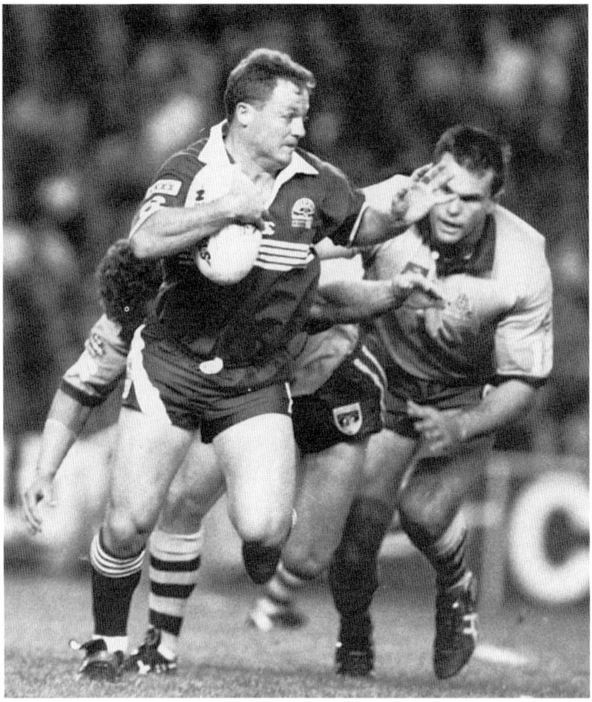

Escaping the clutches of Paul Harragon in a 1994 State of Origin clash.

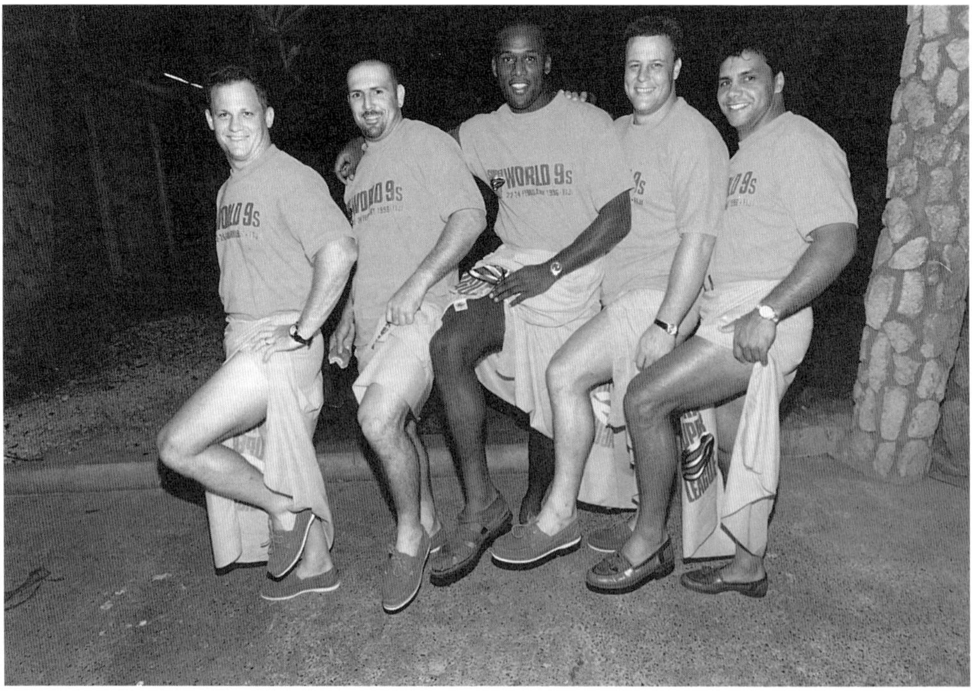


On island time. That's yours truly, Michael Hancock, Wendell Sailor, Glenn Lazarus and Steve Renouf in Fiji for the Super League World Nines competition in 1996.

were flash showponies. We'd proved them wrong, and we had the Winfield Cup to prove it. Queensland Premier Wayne Goss embraced Wayne Bennett. Wally was there to congratulate us, and so were former Broncos and Queensland stars Gene Miles, Lew Platz, Greg Veivers, Mark Murray, John McDonald, Paul McCabe. Nearly an hour after the match ended, we still had not returned to our dressing room. We wanted to make the magic moment last.

On the Broncos' chartered plane back to Brisbane, we players sat upfront together, letting that winning feeling engulf us. At the back of the plane in economy, where the friends and family and VIP supporters sat, the Powers beer flowed. KG and Sandy were back there with Alf's parents, Rita and Harry. Someone asked Mum if she thought Kerrod, Steve and I would be picked in the Australian World Cup squad to play in England, to be named that night. 'They would be if I was a selector,' she declared.

The plane landed at Brisbane and we could not believe our eyes. We'd expected a circus because Brisbane had been mad with excitement all week. People and shops had been decked out in our colours and, incredibly, more than 3000 fans had showed up to watch us at our final training session at Red Hill. It was manic. People had cheered our training drills as if they were the real thing and rock music blasted from the ground's speakers. During the match, some 92 per cent of TV sets in Brisbane were tuned in to the match. But nothing prepared us for the reception awaiting us on grand final night. More than 2000 screaming, cheering supporters were jammed into the airport to welcome us and our trophy home. It was something I never thought I'd see. It was bloody incredible! The masses of people looked like ants from the windows of our plane. On the ground, we were treated like movie stars. We thought there might have been a few people at the airport but you *could not move.* There were people yelling and screaming and hugging us or trying to touch us.

Kim was with me all the way, noisy, laughing, having a ball. The club really looked after all the wives and girlfriends and made them feel special because they know the sacrifices a footy player's partner has to make. The girls have to put up with us being away from home and getting injured, so they deserve to experience the rewards of rugby league as well as its drawbacks. They got as much of a buzz out of our grand final victory as their men did. It's important for clubs to realise that if a player is unhappy off the field there is no way he can perform his best on the field. At the Broncos we have long left behind the old chauvinistic attitudes summed up in low-rent jokes like: 'Did you hear X's wife got hit by a car?' 'Oh really? What was she doin' out of the kitchen?' Wayne, particularly, appreciates the importance of a happy family.

There was more pandemonium at a civic reception in Brisbane's King George Square just after 9 p.m. when Alf led us in a rendition of 'Hey, Hey, We're The Broncos'. (That's the song Alf, Kerrod and I recorded as The Ipswich Connection. It was such a big hit in Australia that some other band called the Monkees ripped it off us, changed the words a bit and sold millions around the world.) Then, as it neared 10 p.m., the fun and frenzy continued at our training ground, Gilbert Park. There were thousands of fans. Many had been there all day, watching the game on a giant screen. They swamped us. They took off Alf's shoes, they took off his socks, they took his cap, and then he dived into the middle of the crowd. I dived right in after him. Alf, Steve Renouf and I crowd-surfed, tumbled over the top of the throng by hundreds of hands. The fans had less luck lifting Lazzo.

From there it was back to the Leagues Club for more celebrating, made even sweeter for me when, with Kerrod and Steve and Broncos Alf, Chris Johns, Willie Carne, Steve Renouf, Mick Hancock and Glen Lazarus, I was picked for the World Cup team. The selectors had obviously consulted Mum. 'Too many good things have been happening to our family lately,' she said when she heard the news, sounding as if there would one day be a reckoning for us Walters getting more than our fair share of good luck. But I'd known I had a chance of being selected after I was picked as a reserve for all three Tests against a spirited Great Britain team when the Poms toured Australia earlier in the year. I'd made it onto the field in each Test in the series, which we won 2–1.

The Broncos players had dinner in a roped-off room – with Wayne, our partners, the club's officials and sponsors. Given my dim memory of the proceedings, I think it was largely a liquid dinner. I think there was a cake fight. I recall throwing cake and rubbing it in Alf's hair. Seems to me his baldness set in right about then. Shirts got ripped and there was wrestling. It was pretty wild. More than 40 kegs and 1800 cartons of beer were sunk that evening – most of it consumed by me, if my sore head for days after was any guide. Brisbane police advised that there was virtually no crime in the city that night, as even crims found grand final partying more fun than breaking the law. We were given buzzcuts by Janine Langer, Lisa Matterson and Sharon Gee, all hairdressers, and had our numbers etched into the back of our heads. Wayne had the letter 'C' for coach cut into his hair. None of us slept for days. We celebrated in one pub after another. On the Wednesday after the grand final we were the stars of a ticker-tape parade through the city, with 20,000 Brisbanites lining the streets five-deep to cheer our motorcade. Lord Mayor Jim Soorley presented us with the keys of the city of Brisbane, and then we set sail on Broncos director Gary Balkin's *Kookaburra Queen* paddle-steamer for a feast of Queensland seafood.

Next day it was the people of Ipswich's chance to turn it on for their hometown boys. Alf, Kerrod and I, and Peter Ryan, Willie Carne and Brett Plowman who had played there as kids, were given a civic reception in front of 10,000 locals. After the reception I motored back to Brisbane, climbed into my monkey suit and, with Kim alongside me and looking fabulous, fronted up for the Broncos presentation night held at the Sir Walter Burnett building at Brisbane

Exhibition Ground. Kerrod was named our player of the year, Gilly best forward and Alf best back. At one late stage of the proceedings, Kerrod, Lazo, Wayne Bennett and I jumped up on stage and 'entertained' the crowd with some songs.

Wayne was in his element, and although he doesn't drink he partied as hard as any of us. But all that week following the grand final, while we were playing up, our coach was also thinking hard about 1993 and our premiership defence. He had a fear that, like Manly in 1987 and Penrith in 1991, we would be one-year wonders. 'Anyone satisfied with the '92 result can forget about playing first grade next season,' he growled. 'There'll be no resting on our laurels.' We were expected back at Red Hill, ready to train, in November.

Wayne thought deeply about our inaugural premiership. He summed it up this way in an article he wrote for *Rugby League Week*:

> Not long ago a rival coach told one of my staff the Broncos couldn't win the premiership because they liked to have a drink and a smoke after games. He'd banned all that. Rugby league was too serious. It's not a big issue, but maybe it sums up a lot of things about the game. How people try to make it too serious, too complex. The reason we're the premiers is because we have a lot of values we haven't lost sight of. I've got a wonderful team who, for five years, have played some great football, football [that] people enjoy watching. And yeah, we have a drink and

smoke . . . well, not me personally. We have fun. We play football like we think it should be played, we approach the game like it should be approached. We put everything in perspective. We realise the competitiveness and professionalism of the business, but at the same time there must be a balance. We've found it at Brisbane, and that is the real reason for our success this season.

Last Sunday was without doubt my greatest moment. I know how much it meant to other people as well as myself. It was a first for the club and it was particularly special to me because I realise I'm probably the first coach who was able to get a football team together from scratch, build them into something I wanted, and win a premiership with them. You recruit them, you develop them, you live with them, you love them, you die for them and then to be able to share the glory with them is something dreams are made of. But I'm no coaching guru. I don't take myself that seriously. Last year we scored 86 tries and conceded 52, this year we scored 87 and conceded 53. Yet last year they all said I couldn't coach and the team couldn't play. We've won a premiership and all of a sudden I'm a better coach and they're a better team. It's such a fine line. Last year we lost many games by two points, this year we won them. Now we're the champions.

Fast-forward now a couple of weeks, to 24 October, for another unforgettable page in my scrapbook. The day and the moment will always be crystal clear. The 1992

World Cup final, Australia versus Great Britain. Kim and our baby son Jack, along with Sandy and KG, were among the 73,631 fans packed into London's Wembley Stadium. Kerrod, who sadly didn't play in the final after he'd been pipped by Steve, had given Mum and Dad the airline tickets he'd won for being the Broncos' player of the year. In the first half, brother Steve was having a blinder as hooker (he would be named man of the match), but I was a reserve on the bench and hurting. The match was tight. Great Britain, with Gary Schofield, Ellery Hanley, Andy Platt, Phil Clarke and Denis Betts, was a formidable outfit and they were giving it to us in a gruelling defensive game. I knew I had something to offer the team and I was itching to get out there and try something and prove my worth to them.

Suddenly, three minutes after halftime, Brad Clyde got injured and came off. 'Get out there, Kevvie,' snapped coach Bob Fulton. My tracksuit was off in a flash and I ran onto the famous pitch. Brad Fittler moved from five-eighth to lock and I slotted in at pivot. Twelve minutes from fulltime, we were down 6–4, their three goals to our two. Time was flying. Something had to be done, and bloody soon. I noticed the English lacked numbers on the blind. Steve Renouf was lurking there. Our eyes met, the move was on. He hit the pedal and ran to the outside of his opposite centre, John Devereux. I hit the gap with a long cut-out pass that we call an out-ball. Steve plucked it out of the air and found himself in open space. He glided the last 20 metres to the line and put the ball down for a try. We were ahead 8–6. Pandemonium erupted. Mal Meninga converted from the sideline. Australia 10 – Great Britain 6. The first time I watched a video of that try I saw a fist-pumping flash of green and gold whizz into the frame and envelop Renouf. The flash, of course, was me.

We call Steve Renouf 'The Pearl' – Ellery Hanley was 'The Black Pearl', Steve's just 'The Pearl'. I loved playing inside him and Chris Johns. Steve can do things on a football field that other champions can only dream about. Kelvin Giles had it right when he said of Steve: 'His acceleration, his balance, his proprioceptability – that is, his ability to know where parts of his body are when they are being tossed and turned in different directions – are outstanding.' In my time as a player, the two most spectacular runners of the ball have been Steve Renouf and Canberra's Brett Mullins. Steve, a family man who is one of 12 kids himself, came to the Broncos as a brilliant attacker with a suspect defence, but he's worked hard on his defensive game. Today he is the complete centre who can set up a try and blot his opposite number out of a game with his tackling – but who still has that lightning speed and flashing feet that can get him around his man and into the clear. Put the glasses down. As he proved in the 1992 grand final and the World Cup final he can turn a game in a twinkle. He's mentally tough, too. Not many blokes could overcome the diabetes condition he has, which at one stage stripped many kilos from his weight, or the physical and psychological effects of the broken jaw he suffered in an off-season incident at his hometown of Murgon in 1993.

The icing on the giant celebration cake that was season 1992 came on 30 October, a week after the World Cup final, when we beat the champion English club side, Wigan, in the World Club Challenge at their home ground, Central Park. It was a fiery match, as their eleven internationals hit our nine head-on. We couldn't believe our eyes when Lazzo ran the ball back from the opening kickoff and Wigan's Andy Platt, one of the very best props in the world, and two other forwards picked him up and drove him backwards. Watching Lazzo being tossed around was frightening. I'm thinking: 'Christ! Here's our big, tough front-rower – *smack!* – they're toying with him like he's a little rag doll! What are we in for here?!' It was then that Andrew Gee, back then an underrated player, came into his own. He realised that we had to hit back hard, and, like a vigilante, singled out their most formidable forward, Platt. Punches flew between them and a violent brawl erupted. From then on, with Wigan out to get square, we ran away with the game, 22–8.

These days, seven years on, Andrew Gee, who turned the tide for us that north-of-England night, is one of the senior guys at the Broncos and relishing the responsibility. He is our forward leader and highly respected in our club. This year, a Brisbane newspaper asked Wayne Bennett who he would like to be stranded with on a desert isle. He said Alf and me, because we would make him laugh, and Gee-Gee because he's such a solid and reliable citizen, and with him on the island we would never starve. Andrew remains a vigilante. It is still his way to pit himself against the best opposing forward and he doesn't often come off second best.

That World Club Challenge game had a funny sidelight. It was a revelation to us that in England you can bet on anything, and one bookmaker had Julian O'Neill 20–1 to score the first try. Not bad odds, considering that Julian is pretty good at scoring tries and was nicknamed 'The Pope' because he refuses to pass the pill. We all bet on him, too, and sure enough in the 17th minute he chimed into the backline, got the ball, and took on their fullback rather than passing to a support. Luckily, he beat his man, scored the opening try and we all got a little richer.

Moments like Steve Renouf's winning try at Wembley and a hundred others as Australia won the World Cup and the Broncos won their first premiership made season 1992 a memorable one. That was the year when, at 25, I felt I had come of age as a player. The player I was then, and am today, evolved from the natural maturing of my footy skills, mental toughness acquired over years of top grade league, and my defined role at the Broncos. If you asked me to describe what kind of player I am, I would say I am a solid team player, rather than a brilliant individual. I've been lucky over the years to have wonderful players inside me and outside me who have helped my game and I feel that I have helped their game as well. My go has always been to back up the brilliant creative players – like Wally, Kerrod and Alf – inside me, and in turn create opportunities for Steve Renouf, Chris Johns, Mick Hancock, Paul Hauff, Willie Carne, Darren Smith, Darren Lockyer, Wendell Sailor and the other fliers outside me. It takes time to know when – and who – to support, when to try something yourself, when to run, pass or kick.

I'm not saying for a minute that blokes like Laurie Daley and Brad Fittler are not team players but they like to do something off their own head, whereas I tend to play in conjunction with someone else. Maybe that's why Alf generally has played his best football for the Broncos. He and I work as a unit, his brilliance and my team play are complementary, but when Alf is paired in Tests with another brilliant individualist in Laurie or Brad there is not the same combination. I don't think a player like Alf and a player like Laurie fit cohesively in the same side because they are so similar and sometimes jar each other's game. Ricky Stuart, however, like me a team player, and Laurie – or Brad – go together like clockwork. Cohesion is vital if a half-back–five-eighth pairing is to be effective, because the halves handle the ball more than anyone else on the field except the dummy half.

When I played in the juniors at Ipswich I was a specialist halfback, but some little blond bloke had a mortgage on the No. 7 jersey in the rep teams so I was happy to become a five-eighth. A halfback, generally, can afford to be play his own game, while the five-eighth must be the link between the forwards and the outside backs. There are always exceptions, but that's the way my game has developed. Anyhow, that's the way I see myself as a player. And you play to your strengths. I like getting the ball in my hands at second receiver then sharing it around. I've got good vision on the field, and can work out where the opposition's numbers are down and who their weak links are, and direct play accordingly. I take wrong options, like everyone else, but mostly over the years I've got it right.

I believe in muscle memory, and because I've been playing since I was a kid and have acquired a big knowledge bank, a lot of what I do on the field I do instinctively. I've been taught over the years that what I practise at training each week is what I will do on Sunday. I've also learned that when I try too hard to make things happen I come unstuck. If I relax and let my muscle memory take over, if I just go with the flow, I have a much better game. It is no coincidence that I had my best year in rugby league in 1998. What with Kim's illness, and worrying about my family, there were so many other things occupying my mind that I scarcely gave footy a thought. I just went out there each week and did it. It diverted me from my grief. I didn't worry about my form, the opposition, whether I'd make the Origin team – and everything fell into place on the field.

I thank the Broncos kicking coach Graham McColm for helping me with my kicking game. Early in my career, I considered that kicking was just giving the ball away cheaply to the opposition and it was never part of my game, but now I know that, done right, kicking is a potent attacking weapon. Graham has an Aussie Rules background and because of his tuition I now go into a game knowing that I can usually kick the ball where I want to kick it. Long kicks to gain ground, bombs on the opposition tryline – once that ball's in the air, it's anyone's – kicks to put pressure on a shaky opponent, kicks to trap the opposition behind their goal-line, chips, grubbers . . . Instead of as it was in the old days when I'd get kicks right two times out of ten, these days I get them right 70–80 per cent of the time. At the Broncos, Alf (before he retired), Darren Lockyer, Ben Walker, Michael Devere, me – all the kickers spend lots of time practising that part of our repertoire. We've seen Darren's kicking improve over the years, and Alf's too. Early in his career, Alf couldn't kick the ball out of sight on a dark night but through practice he became a master.

I like to think my defence has improved, even though I don't go along with people over the years who've said my tackling is suspect. Reporters started saying that my defence was lousy after that one bad game against Brad Izzard in 1990 and it became accepted wisdom that I couldn't defend. For a while, and in weaker moments, I believed what they said. I hadn't been monstered by Brad before that semi-final, and I never was again, but I used my shocker to brush up on my technique. Big Brett Plowman, brother Kerrod and Trevor Gillmeister took me out to the sand-pit at training and knocked my defence into shape. If you don't tackle Brett correctly he'll kill you. Gilly's defence was always his strongest point. They called him

The Axe and his tackles hurt you so much that his defence was a form of attack. Nowadays I work constantly on defence with Peter Ryan and Tonie Carroll. Wayne Bennett has always drummed into me that everyone playing football at the level we are is capable of tackling – you just have to apply yourself to it. Still, some days there's just nothing you can do. Some days guys are always going to run over the top of you.

There have been times when misconceptions about my tackling have helped the Broncos. In successive grand finals against St George in 1992 and 1993, their coach Brian Smith targeted me and Alf by having his huge runners Scott Gourley and Tony Priddle charge at us all day. It didn't work. Although we were smaller, we brought the big blokes down time and again. I think they only got the odd ball away after we'd taken them on. My brother Steve, who hooked at Canberra for years, told me Tim Sheens always had his biggest, fastest Raiders run repeatedly at Alf, me and Steve Renouf. But it wasn't because he didn't think we could tackle. He'd singled us out as potent attackers and thought he could sap our energy by making us work overtime in defence. We'd have huge tackle counts, and if you see a back with a tackle count up in the 20s it's a safe bet he's been tagged as a danger man.

There are not many unfilled pages in my scrapbook after a lifetime in league, but, after all is said and done, I've learned that the difference between a good game and a bad game is only a couple of beers! Sometimes you walk off the field and you think: 'Christ, I was woeful!' But come nine or ten o'clock at night, after a few drinks, you're convinced you were the best player on the field. And why not? I don't want to give myself too much of a rap, but since we're on the subject here's how two men who have my greatest respect rate my game.

Wally Lewis, when he was asked to contribute a few memories and opinions for this book, said: 'Kevin's importance to the Broncos' success mustn't be underestimated. When Kevvie and Alf lead from the front, everyone else follows [Wally was speaking days before Alf retired in April, 1999]. They have built the side around those two players, similar to how the West Indies rally around Brian Lara. When Lara performs, the others around him lift, and when Kevin and Alf are firing, so are the Broncos. The Broncos have achieved success because they have been a stable unit and have made minimal changes. Kevin and Alf have been rock solid as a halves combination.'

And Wayne Bennett once summed up my game this way: 'Kevvie is always the life of the team, but when it comes to football he's really serious and a terrific competitor. He's a magnificent team player who would rather play badly and the team play well, than be a star and the team play badly.' I guess that's true. My team and my team-mates are important to me. I have a thing about not ever letting them down. For instance, I'm never late for games or training or club functions. I'm late for everything else in my life, always late dropping the kids off at school, rushing here and there because I'm behind time. But for football, I'm never late.

I just love playing footy. I owe the game an enormous

amount. I've made lifelong friends and have a treasure chest of memories. I have been well paid and my loved ones and I enjoy a good lifestyle because of this game that I play. All this, but I'd play for nothing. To be very well rewarded for doing something I love is a bonus.

If there's anything I could change, it's that I've paid too much attention to critics over the years. I'm one of those players who *do* read the papers and take to heart what journalists write about me. I know I shouldn't, but there you go. When they said I couldn't tackle, for a while I doubted myself even though I knew there was nothing much wrong with my defence. When they said I was out of my depth in State of Origin I almost believed them, but time has proved that I can cut it in the maroon jumper. Sometimes I've gone onto the field with the critics' words ringing in my ears and determined to prove the bastards wrong.

Take that Origin series in 1992. Wally Lewis had retired in 1991 and Origin I was my first game as first choice five-eighth. I was a bundle of nerves before the game. 'Club football is one thing. State of Origin is something completely different,' I told writer Mike Colman in an interview and photo shoot before the game. 'When it comes to State of Origin, Wally has been the King. He's been the King for so long, no one can ever really take his place. You can only play your best and be yourself.' Queensland manager Dick 'Tosser' Turner, who was with us, helped me out. 'No question, the influence of Wally is still here. But it's better to look at it this way: Kevin Walters' ability has won him the coveted five-eighth role which was made available with Wally's retirement. For over ten years that jumper was Wally's. There were others who wore it, but it was never theirs. They were fill-ins because he wasn't available and as soon as he came back it was there waiting for him. Well, he's not coming back this time, and Kevin has done very well to win his spot.' Speaking to Colman, I added: 'I've been a great admirer of Wally's for years, but you have to get on with things. That was our first training run without Wally today and we seemed to go OK. Life goes on.'

After the interview the photographer thought it would be amusing if he took a picture of me wearing a crown and posing as the new King. I said: 'No way!'

We lost Origin I 14–6 to a great Blues team. Their forwards – Lazarus, Elias, Harragon, Cartwright, Sironen, Clyde – got over the top of ours, who found it tough going to build an attacking platform for the backs. We were on the back foot, but even so my team-mates voted me their player's player. Yet, for Origin II and III, I was dumped to the bench. It seemed unfair. We won the second match 5–4 and lost the third 16–4. After that, it was bloody good to get back to the Broncos.

Alf Langer and I were partners in crime for a long time. We go back, one way or another, nearly 20 years. Before his bombshell retirement, he was what the Broncos are all about. It's been said before, but over the past decade there wasn't a better footballer in the game. He was the heart and soul of Brisbane. There were times when I was immensely envious of his talent and what he achieved in the game. His breathtaking skills and leadership made him a legend. In attack, there was no more dangerous player. If his speed and footwork didn't break the defence, he'd bust through with his amazing strength (he was incredibly strong even as a kid). Or he'd pull a superb kick out of his bag of tricks and beat you that way. His options were many and he was a master of them all. A measure of Alf is the number of club and Origin matches and Tests that he won on his own.

Alf was great for my career. We conjured up over many years an eerily instinctive combination. We always knew what the other had on his mind and on a day when we were both firing, scheming behind a dominant pack, we were able to control the game, our passes and kicks sticking like glue. We made our own luck. On one memorable occasion at Cronulla we were down by two in the final moments, when Alf chipped ahead and followed on. Instead of trying to pick the ball up, he went to toe it over the Sharks' try-line, but miscued and connected with his instep. The ball shot forwards, way too fast and hard, and looked certain to go over the dead-ball line. But centimetres this side of it, the ball landed on its point, spun outrageously backwards and somehow stopped dead, barely in the field of play. A complete fluke. When Alf chips, you need your head examined if you don't chase. I did just that and was there to fall on the stationary ball and score the winning try. When people congratulated us on our carefully choreographed try, we didn't bother putting them straight, just grinned and silently thanked our lucky stars. Alf and I motivated each other. There was always a bit of on-field chat going on between us, one revving the other up, saying, 'Well done,' when things worked out and 'Come on, mate, let's give it to 'em' when they didn't.

Alf was a fine captain. He had great confidence in his own ability and in his team-mates. So he never panicked when things looked bleak. That's one of the reasons why often we could come from way behind to win a game. Other teams knew never to relax against a side with Alf in it. A miracle pass to put one of us into a gap, a chip with nothing on that ends in a try, a solo tackle-busting burst: Alfie could do it all. He certainly kept his head. When we'd be blowing up over a bad decision, Alf could calm us down and get our minds back on the game. He was also a master at gamesmanship and thought nothing of pushing a referee to the limit if it meant getting an advantage for his team.

All that, and he's funny and a decent bloke to boot. Alf was always being hassled big-time in his playing days. Everyone thought they owned him. Kids, parents, anyone and everyone all wanted to be near him or to touch him. He always handled himself magnificently in spite of a lot of aggravation. He never failed to give an autograph when fans demanded one and always spoke politely, even when people weren't polite to him. Strangers would come up to him and *biff, biff, biff,* they'd prod him in the stomach and dig him in the back. 'Langer, give us an autograph!' they'd demand. 'Langer, you're pretty good for a little man!' He'd simply turn, grin calmly and do what they asked without fuss. (Wally was another who copped a bad time from the fans, but he wasn't always able to put up with the invasion of privacy and sometimes said what was on his mind.)

Alf always gladly gave me advice, and was there to talk about problems on and off the field. His humour lifted you up. Just when you thought the world was coming down on you, he'd say or do something funny and you couldn't help but laugh. He's been a good friend to me for a lot of years and he will continue to be now that he's retired. He's never been afraid to have a dig at me, like when he demanded 10 weeks' rent in 1990, and when he defused an uncomfortable situation that arose when Wayne was considering both Alf and me to succeed Gene Miles as Broncos captain in 1991. We both knew Alf would get the job, of course, and he did get it, but until the day he retired he'd gee me up: 'You know, Kevvie, *you* could have been the captain of this joint . . . you missed it by *that* much . . .' He kept my spirits up during Broncos and State of Origin disappointments. And I'll cherish forever the strength he gave me through his friendship when Kim got sick, and after she died.

For all his goodheartedness and happy-go-lucky ways, when it came to football Alf was totally ruthless in his determination to get an advantage over opponents. That's what made him a champion. He changed the game of rugby league. The ARL brought in a law to ban his tackling style, where he'd use a leg and a throw to bring an attacker crashing down. 'It just developed from tackling bigger blokes. It was an easier way to bring a bigger bloke down,' he said. And Alf's upper-body strength and low centre of gravity enabled him to prise the ball from the grasp of the most powerful opponent, so administrators scurried to rewrite the rule books to outlaw his ball-stealing.

Alf was a hardhead, and he was fearless. Against Cronulla in 1997, big prop Les Davidson, feared and respected as the hardest man in rugby league, dragged Alf off the ball in a turnover. But reputations meant nothing to Alf and he whacked Davo with a haymaker. Davo hit back with a ferocious combination. 'It didn't look good,' Davidson said of the mismatch. 'But if it happened again and someone threw a punch at me, I'd have to do the same thing. The saving grace was that nobody was hurt. I have to give Alf his due because he went straight into an in-close fighting style and tied me up. He's a very tough, strong little bloke.' After the match, Alf was boasting to everyone who'd listen about his pugilistic prowess. He swore that as the blue raged and the punches were flying he kept instructing Davo to keep his right hand up.

CHAPTER SIX

# IN THE BRONCOS' STABLE

At the Broncos the players and partners see a bit of each other outside footy. Part of it is that most of us get on naturally; part of it is that our club fosters a family feeling. I'm not saying other clubs aren't close and I'm not qualified to talk about other outfits, but I do know that I've never seen a club so close as the Broncos. When Kim was ill, nothing was too much trouble for the management as they did everything in their power to ease our pain. Wayne and my team-mates and their wives or girlfriends were so loving towards Kim and supported me and our sons through all the dark days. I had wives bringing meals over to our house and offering to look after the children. I was allowed to bring the boys to training if I couldn't find a babysitter. I'll never be able to repay everyone for the support they gave us. It might be great to be a Queenslander but it's even better to be a Bronco. This season, 1999, is my tenth with the club. As I write this book, only Mick Hancock, that wonderful, angry, wholehearted, hyperactive winger – surely no player in the game hates being tackled as much as Mick – has been there longer, now that Alf's gone. I've played well over 200 games in the maroon, yellow and white.

At the moment, as I write this in May 1999, the Broncos are not having things our own way, though we think we'll be there at season's end. But this season apart, and with the exception of periodic lows over the years, we have one of the proudest records in rugby league. In the eleven seasons from 1988, our first year in the premiership, until the end of 1998, we won the grand final four times: in 1992, '93, '97 (the Super League Telstra Cup) and '98. We were club champions in '92 and '96. Twenty-four Broncos have played for Australia, and we provided Test skippers Wally and Alf. Each year Broncos are the bulk of the Queensland State of Origin team. Wayne Bennett, the best coach I've ever had, as both strategist and motivator, has coached Queensland and Australia. Sure, he has always had a team of champions to work with at Brisbane, but how many times do we see a team of champions not come up to scratch as a champion team?

Wayne's achievement has been to harness the talents of his players to create a side, greater than the sum of our individual parts, that plays an adventurous, spectacular, rolling and lightning-fast brand of rugby league. To the Broncos, field goals are a cop-out unless it's to break a deadlock, and we often take a tap from a penalty to keep up the pressure rather than kick for touch or go for goal. We can score tries from deep in our half. We are known as a team that takes risks – long passes in our own territory, speculator kicks early in the tackle count – teams have learned to expect the unexpected from us. But there's nothing unplanned or haphazard about the way we play. What looks spontaneous on the field is the result of years of skill drills. Wayne has always paid attention to the basic ingredients of rugby league: passing, kicking, speed, agility, strength, support play, tackling. Often we are behind early in a game but come roaring back. As ex-Bronco Glenn Lazarus said after we'd beaten his Melbourne Storm in 1998: 'With 15 minutes to go it was 12-all, but the Broncos do everything with precision and never panic. We blinked twice, relaxed for a second or two and suddenly they were 12 points in front of us.'

We may be crowd-pleasers on the field but, apart from putting in the hard work at training, our good record is founded on pragmatism. We've never been allowed to get big-headed or take success for granted. 'We're vulnerable,' Wayne has always drummed into us. 'We have achieved what everyone has wanted most, and success is a terrific feeling, but we have to be careful that things don't change. If just one or two players lose their hunger, get carried away with the achievement or become selfish and think they are better than their mates, we are back where we started.' He explained to *Rugby League Week*'s Tony Durkin in 1993:

> In our five years in the competition, we have won more games than any other club, so we have been consistently winning for a long time. But it has been a learning process for everyone here – and a slow one at that. We have had to grasp important things like discipline, reducing unforced errors, combating our tough travel program and the grind of 22 weeks of tough footy. A lot of people here have had to change their ways, and some took longer than others. We were being beaten in crucial matches, but most times I thought we were beating ourselves. I tried most things, including fining players. And then all of a sudden this season, it clicked. Not just 10 or 11 of them realised what was needed, but the entire squad of 20. When this happened, I knew we had a team.

Wayne confessed back in that premiership year that he was disappointed at not winning the premiership in the Broncos' first year, 1988, but came to understand that 'players like Allan Langer, Kerrod Walters and Gene Miles had to learn certain aspects of the game, despite the fact they were all seasoned rep players. It was a different ball game. Kerrod, for instance, was a marvellously skilled player, but his mistake rate was alarming. We used numbers with him, limiting his mistakes to, say, five a game, and we worked down from there. Now I'm pleased to say that Kerrod is just about a mistake-free player who has had his best season, but it takes time.'

We've also set the pace off the field. We were the first privately owned club and, like it or not, our progressive thinking and embrace of modern sports marketing concepts has changed the game forever and dragged rugby league into the world of sports professionalism. From the day the Broncos hung out their shingle, our smart, hardheaded management have set new standards in rugby league. They acquired a great coaching staff and some of the best players in the game, paid them well and gave them a setup in which they could perform at their best. The benefits of being a Bronco are many, but as in any successful business there's no such thing as a free lunch. The bottom line is always there to keep us focused. For us, that line is winning games and drawing sponsors and fans through the gates. Players considered unsuitable – and that can be because of poor form, advancing age, misbehaviour, disruptiveness or an inability to get on with team-mates – are shown the door.

One price we pay for success is that we are unpopular with followers of other teams who may envy our success. A victory over the Broncos is always especially sweet. Maybe it's the tall poppy syndrome in action. Maybe it's the win-at-all-costs attitude of our players like Wally, Alf, Lazzo and Gorden Tallis – not to mention the stern attitude that Wayne Bennett often adopts in public and his inability to suffer fools gladly – that puts us offside.

It seems we have always been at loggerheads with

the League establishment. Five weeks into season 1988, we were blueing with them because we insisted on displaying our sponsor Power Brewing's banners at Lang Park even though XXXX had advertising sign rights at the ground. We complained bitterly that the rule that banned State of Origin selections from playing for their club in the lead-up to the interstate game victimised us because the ruling usually deprived us of up to 10 of our players when other clubs lost about three tops. We took on the League when we thought we were entitled to a better compensation deal on our heavy travel costs. We believed we deserved to have a semi-final or final played in Brisbane and said so. We were bitterly critical when we thought the judiciary was picking on us, especially over Alf's tackling style and a number of heavy suspensions they dealt to Kerrod. We seemed to be constantly at war with the New South Wales Rugby League. We refused to let them stand over us. We bucked when NSWRL general manager John Quayle announced that there would be an investigation into our finances because we were suspected of rorting the salary cap then in force. He accused us of having a 'screw everyone else' attitude. There was definitely a feeling down south of 'There they go again, the whingeing bloody Broncos'. A siege mentality set in at our club, a feeling of us against them, that bound us together and made us stronger. It's probably true that our treatment at the hands of the League establishment was the trigger for Super League and led us to embrace a more enlightened way of running the game.

The Broncos have got a lot of critics but, let's face it, they do things right. Recruitment has always been a strong point, and our talent scouts haven't been wrong too often. We've snapped up established players such as Glenn Lazarus, Trevor Gillmeister, Dale Shearer, Peter Jackson, Sam Backo, Chris Johns, Gorden Tallis, Darren Smith and Anthony Mundine, but our go has mainly been to see the potential in young unknowns and turn them into champions. Julian O'Neill was first spotted as a 15-year-old playing for St Brendan's, Yeppoon. Michael Hancock was 17 and playing for Toowoomba in the State League when he impressed our scouts. Alan Cann was a 16-year-old kid at Beenleigh High. Steve Renouf, Wendell Sailor and Andrew Gee were others signed from school. Willie Carne was playing in the Under-19s in Roma. Terry Matterson and Gavin Allen were reserve graders at Eastern Suburbs and St George. I was not exactly setting the league world on fire when Wayne brought me up from Canberra. Now, as the new millennium approaches, and the stars of the 1990s near the end of their careers, a new breed of Bronco is being blooded. In 1999, Shane Webcke, a Bronco discovery, is already a Test player. Such future stars as Kevin Campion, Phil Lee, Tonie Carroll, Michael Devere, Petero Civoniceva and the Walker brothers are now making their mark, and are living proof of our management's astute recruiting.

People say we have a vast area to draw our players from, and that's true, but the fact is that if a number of clubs including the Broncos are out to sign up a promising bloke, nine times out of ten the kid will become a Bronco. We have a reputation for nurturing our young players and making them feel at home. Parents like their sons to play with us because we don't have some of the problems that other clubs do. We encourage the younger Broncos to go to university or do an apprenticeship so they are occupied while they're not training. Kids who are bored and have plenty of money tend to get into trouble. When young men, like Darren Lockyer, come from the bush to Brisbane, the Broncos place them with a family in a home where they have responsibilities rather than stick them in a home unit on their own and say: 'Here's $200 a week to live on . . . see ya at trainin'.'

We've also got hardheaded businessmen in the club who can counsel players about investments and help them hang onto their money. 'No work, no play' is the go at our club. Our founding chairman Barry Maranta's pledge was to try to ensure that players left the Broncos not only better footballers but better people, with skills that would help them earn money for the rest of their lives. We are encouraged to do media work but also earn a buck in a trade or business. For a while I worked with MMI Insurance, drumming up third party business for the car fleets of Broncos sponsors. The Broncos management help us make money, but also try to stop us from losing it. They do their best to protect players from the hordes of smarties out there trying to fleece footy stars. Some player managers fit this description. I haven't got a lot of time for football managers. I think too many leech off players' money. My manager Barry Collins is an honourable exception.

I'm one who has benefited from being a Bronco. I've gone from being a boy to a man in my time with the club. For that, in so many ways, I thank Wayne Bennett. He's my coach, and he can be ruthless (ask Wally, or Alan Cann or Kerrod or Julian O'Neill who he was forced to cut from the club), but he's also a friend. He has been like a second father to me. He's never failed to give me advice and put me on the right track. Tell him something in confidence and it stays with him. I trust and respect him. He's a great role model to a young bloke. He doesn't drink or smoke but enjoys life as much as anyone who does. I'm sure he has faults, but I can't think of too many. He can be intimidating and brutally honest and is not afraid of hurting your feelings. He says: 'If I stop harassing you, I stop caring about you.' He also has no interest in being popular and doesn't run away from making hard decisions. He cut Wally from the club when Wally was the biggest player in the game, and he was responsible for Kerrod leaving when he thought my brother had reached his use-by date. Nothing personal, just part of his job. Wayne knows there can be no room for sentiment.

He terrorises the media. He must have had some bad experiences with reporters early in his career. The saying goes that rugby league needs the media, but I don't think Wayne agrees with that. He believes that certain sections of the media have not always given the Broncos a fair go, and he puts so much of his heart into us that he takes criticism very personally. In private, he's warm and funny and very wise, but the public knows Wayne as an austere, unsmiling fellow. It's not often he opens up to the press, but once to journalist Steve Crawley he explained that he never wanted a public profile. He said he coached because he relished the challenge. He was uncomfortable in the public eye. 'I've never been accused of being the life of the party, but that doesn't mean I don't enjoy a good time. To me a good time is hanging around guys like Alfie and the Walters twins. I mean, being around those guys is a lot of fun. Something's always happening. They don't take life too seriously and they certainly don't take themselves seriously. Being such a character is not something that sits comfortably with me, personally. I see a sense of spirit and excitement in those guys I'd like to have myself. But if I did, I probably wouldn't be coach.'

Other key Broncos staffers are the kicking coach Graham McColm who taught us all how to kick in general play and turned Darren Lockyer into a fine goalkicker, the strength coach Dan Baker, conditioners Steve Nance and Craig Bellamy, and trainer and conditioner Kelvin Giles when he was with us. Kelvin was a strength coach at Canberra and followed Wayne north. He brought a real air of professionalism to the Broncos. He, as much as anyone, had a lot to do with our premiership wins in 1992 and 1993. A lot of guys found him very confrontational, but I never had a problem with Kelvin. I always found him approachable and incredibly knowledgeable. He could talk to you about anything from the First World War to obscure events at the Olympic Games. He's been to every Games since 1956.

You never say never, but it's hard to imagine some of the incidents involving booze and bad behaviour that have made headlines at other clubs this season happening at the Broncos. We've had the odd problem over the years with players who go off the rails, but bringing the club into disrepute just ain't tolerated at Brisbane. Our management and Wayne will help a player with personal problems, but they're not stupid and if the bloke won't help himself he's history. Ask Julian O'Neill. Julian was talked about as the next Wally Lewis when he was coming through the Broncos ranks. It didn't happen and he only has himself to blame. When he's sober he's a perfect gentleman who would give you the shirt off his back. But as with all of us, alcohol changes you. I know – I've done some lunatic things on the grog. Julian and swimming champ Samantha Riley could have been Australia's golden sporting couple. I remember the day they met. She was having breakfast in the restaurant of a big hotel in Sydney and the Broncos were there too. Julian's and Sam's eyes met, and you could see the spark. We all thought . . . but for one reason or another it didn't work out. Julian got in some strife up here; the club tried to help him out as much as it could. Wayne saved his arse a few times, but Julian had to go, for better or worse. A lot of the clubs he moved on to tried to help him too – Perth, the London Broncos, now Souths. As late as early 1999 he was still finding himself in trouble, although he seems to have made a real effort to pull himself together after a notorious motel incident. He's had a lot of wake-up calls, Julian. Until he truly admits he's got a problem with the drink, his life won't change – he'll continue to get into trouble. Julian's still young and hopefully smart enough to do something about it, but unless he does he'll never be the footballer he could be.

Not that we don't know how to enjoy ourselves at the Broncos. As Alf once put it to Tony Durkin in a *Rugby League Week* feature on our club: 'We let our hair down after a win, but what's wrong with that? We train hard and play hard, and maybe we party too hard, too. But we do it together, as mates, and we enjoy all of it. I don't doubt that's been one of the secrets of our success. We practise our skills over and over again, to the stage where we have confidence in ourselves and our mates. We love to go out there and throw the ball about. Within reason, we can do anything we like on the field. Ask anyone who plays league and they'll tell you there's no better feeling than scoring a length-of-the-field try, particularly when seven or eight guys have handled the ball.'

When Trevor Gillmeister and Glenn Lazarus came to our club we got serious. For many years there was a perception that the Broncos could be beaten through the forwards. Belt us and we'd buckle, people said. That was rubbish, but there's no doubt that after Gilly joined in 1991 and Lazzo in 1992, no one accused us of being soft any more. He was as solid as Uluru for us, giving us driving go-forward with his powerful hit-ups and making our ruck defence hard and uncompromising. The sight of Glenn taking the ball from the kickoff and storming 30 metres upfield and punching holes in the opposition gave us all a surge of confidence. He was never a guy who ranted and raved about how tough he was, but ask other props about Lazzo and they'll tell you he was *very* tough. Each year at Origin time, when he represented New South Wales against us, we got a fresh appreciation of the guy's quality.

Early on, though, Glenn could be a grumpy bugger off the field. He was a worrier and seemed ground down by life's responsibilities. Enter Wayne. After we'd had a couple of lean seasons in 1995 and 1996 he pulled us all aside and gave us straight his assessment of each of us, not just as players, but as men. He was concerned about our attitude to people and life. He sat down with Lazzo and told him to lighten up. As Glenn told reporter Tony Durkin: 'I got the message from a few people that being "Mr Grump" didn't exactly help my cause, and I wasn't exactly fostering a warm feeling with everyone in the Broncos camp. I made a conscious effort to be a kinder, less intense person. Without going into the nitty gritty of what transpired in the room that day, let's just say that Wayne told me he believed I could be a nicer person to have around the place. He has a way about him, of telling people things, and getting the message across. When I thought about it, I realised he was right.'

Wayne always sticks up for his men when he knows it's warranted. He certainly stood by Kerrod when my brother was going through a horror patch in 1994. That was his year to forget. He was struck down by pneumonia and viral meningitis which caused shocking headaches. Not surprisingly, his form suffered. 'Without doubt, this was my worst season ever,' Kerrod grumbled. He also copped it from the judiciary. He was sent off twice and suspended. All hell broke loose when he decked Saints' Tony Priddle with a high tackle. Kerrod was suspended for a month and fined $5000 by the NSWRL for bringing the game into disrepute. Kerrod's tackle was a ball-and-all job on a much taller player. He leapt up and no doubt caught Priddle high, but there was no hard impact with Tony's head, and there was no malice in the tackle. From the time he was a kid, Kerrod has never been a nasty player and his judiciary record pretty much backs that up. But the NSWRL judiciary outed him for four weeks, and when Kerrod demanded to know what he was guilty of – was it intentional, reckless or careless behaviour? – he was told it was none of his business. Kerrod blew up. He accused the NSWRL of victimising him because he was a Bronco.

Wayne blew up too over the unfair treatment of his player. He went public in *Rugby League Week*, making a scathing attack on Kerrod's persecutors. 'Consistency and commonsense is all I've ever asked of the judiciary,' he fumed. Warming up, he continued:

> The four-week suspension handed down to Kerrod Walters has enraged me. And this is not just the issue of a coach sticking up for one of his players.

Every guy in my club and all those who saw the incident on TV know Kerrod did not deserve four weeks for the tackle on Tony Priddle . . . Kerrod's tackle was high, I am not disputing that. But after viewing the video of the incident many times, I can't be sure whether contact was made with the chest, the neck or the chin. What I can be certain of, though, is that there was absolutely no malice in the tackle. The arm making contact with the player was not stiff, nor was his fist clenched . . .

This, of course, is the same judiciary that just a few weeks earlier found Canberra's Brett Mullins not guilty of a high tackle. And when the two incidents are compared, Mullins' tackle appeared to be twice as bad and, without question, higher . . . On that evidence, that panel could not find Kerrod guilty and exonerate Mullins. By doing so, they have shown gross inconsistency in their verdicts. In fact, I would like the panel to explain the difference to me, and I'm prepared to fly to Sydney any time to hear their rationale. Even though the injustice done to the player in this incident riles me, and the lack of commonsense and the inconsistency annoys me, what has really got my back up is the fact the judiciary chairman refused to tell Kerrod what he was guilty of . . . Twice he was informed he would not be told. And that is a denial of natural justice. To close this sorry saga, Kerrod now has no right of appeal. That may have been satisfactory years ago when players were playing for peanuts, but not when they are professionals.

Wayne can be ruthless. He knows champions can't play on forever, and when a man, no matter how great he has been for us in the past prime, begins to slow down, there is no place for him with the Broncos. There may be no harder job for a coach than to have to tell a player he likes and respects to look elsewhere for a game. The bell tolls for us all, but that doesn't make it easier when your number is up. And the break is more traumatic in a club that fosters close friendships, as ours does.

Trevor Gillmeister had been an inspiration to us. He was smaller than the usual forward, but his heart was as big as Queensland and he had a peerless tackling technique. He missed very few games through injury in spite of the pounding he put his body through each game. In his three years with us we won two premierships and he was recalled to the Queensland Origin side. He was brutal on the field, a hard, hard man, but after hours he was a great mate who really knew how to enjoy himself. Gilly got cut at the end of 1993. Wayne told him that, as a bloke getting on in years, he couldn't be retained under the salary cap. To keep him, he was told, would mean cutting a couple of younger forwards. 'Some tough decisions have to be made in the game these days, and letting Trevor go ranks among the hardest this club has had to make in six years,' said Wayne. Gilly took it on the chin, but was emotional. 'This is home, this is where my friends are, this is my future,' he said. 'If I had the choice I'd be staying, but the Broncos made it so I didn't have a choice.' The fans loved him as much as his team-mates and 500 turned up to a farewell lunch just before the grand final in 1993. Letters and cards of support also poured in. Gilly proposed a truce between the Broncos and his new club, the Penrith Panthers, when we played each other the following year. Knowing Gilly, he was not serious. His performances for us in the games after he knew he was on the way out were the measure of the man. It must have been sweet revenge when he played three Tests for Australia against the Kiwis, in 1995. The Broncos' 1993 premiership was a tribute to Trevor Gillmeister.

Before the grand final, though, there was a State of Origin series, and Tests against the Kiwis. If ever an Origin series summed up my problems with the Queensland selectors, it was 1993. I approached the series on a high. After the Broncos thrashed Penrith in April, Wayne Bennett gave me a wrap: 'If there is a better five-eighth playing in any country, I haven't seen him. If I was Queensland coach, I wouldn't have anyone else there. I know I keep pushing Kevvie's barrow, but I think his teammates would tell you the same thing. His creativity and the space he gives his outside men, which is the role of the five-eighth, are unequalled in the game. His running game was right back today.' Alf Langer added: 'I want Kevin at five-eighth for Origin, and I don't mind saying it.' In the first match, Laurie Daley and Ricky Stuart outplayed Alf and me and in a hard defensive game. They won 14–10 at Lang Park. This was the match where

Channel 9 broadcast an X-rated pep talk from our skipper Mal Meninga as we grouped in the centre of the field before the kickoff. This wasn't the last time prying cameras embarrassed a Queenslander in 1993. So often in State of Origin, the team winning the first clash has dropped the second, leading to a spinetingling decider in the third match. No such luck this year. In Origin II, New South Wales beat us 16–12 at Sydney Football Stadium to wrap up the series. It was close. We led 6–0 at halftime but, as they always do, the Blues roared back. They were leading 16–6 with 11 minutes to go when I scored a try, which Dale Shearer converted: 16–12 to New South Wales. With seconds to go, Mal broke clear and tore 40 metres upfield. Laurie Daley collared him and Mal passed to Mark Hohn who was in support, but the ball went loose. The series was gone. I was happy with my game in that second match against the Blues, especially pleased that I'd managed to turn the tables on Laurie. My team-mates voted me player's player. So why wouldn't I be mighty disappointed when the selectors dropped me to the bench for Origin III at Lang Park? Julian O'Neill took my position. It was heartening when Australian coach Bob Fulton spoke out. 'After watching Kevin's performances in the first two games,' said Bozo, 'the decision has left many people shaking their heads in disbelief.'

Funny how things turn out, though. The game – it was a dead rubber and I wasn't even in the run-on team – promised little, but it turned out to be one I'll never forget. Modesty prevents me from crowing about how I proved the selectors wrong, so I'll pass you over to the match report in the League's yearbook:

> The turning point came at halftime when, trailing 12–8, Queensland coach Wally Lewis replaced five-eighth Julian O'Neill with Kevin Walters. O'Neill, thrown into the hotseat in his Origin debut, endured a difficult first half before Lewis opted to replace him with the more experienced Walters. The move signalled a dramatic turnaround for the Maroons, who began to show greater cohesion from the beginning of the second half. The break came midway through the second half when Dale Shearer, Willie Carne, Allan Langer, Mark Coyne and Kevin Walters were all involved in a movement which led to a try to Steve Walters. Minutes later, Lindner crashed through tackles by Tim Brasher and Ricky Stuart to score a well-deserved try which gave Queensland a lead of 20–12. Then a Kevin Walters kick produced a second try for Carne 10 minutes from fulltime . . .

Wally explained why he had brought me on at halftime: 'I just thought Kevvie and Alf would give us the combination we seemed to be lacking. Those two could play together blindfolded.' The action wasn't confined to football. Steve and Benny Elias belted each other in the scrums, and one flare-up in the 23rd minute led to an all-in brawl with Steve and Benny whaling away and Martin Bella and Paul Harragon singling each other out for a heavyweight bout.

I was selected for the Australian team that played the Kiwis in New Zealand, and made the run-on side for the First Test. With Mal Meninga unavailable because of a club match suspension, my five-eighth rivals Laurie Daley and Brad Fittler played in the centres. Unfortunately for me, when Mal returned for the Second and Third Tests he claimed his centre spot, Laurie got my No. 6 jersey and I saw out the remaining two Tests from the bench. Shades of what happened at Canberra in 1987. Still, it was good to be part of Australia's 3–0 series whitewash.

Before the 1993 grand final against St George, Wayne gathered us together with a grave look on his face. He said that someone he knew in the St George camp had given him a copy of Saints' game plan and tip sheet. At training he read from the document he said had been secretly passed on to him. On it was every Bronco, 1 to 17, and beside our name was Saints' opinion of our ability. 'Kevin Walters,' he read out. 'Good hands, quick off the mark, not strong defensively on the left side. Along with Langer and his brother Kerrod, known as the Ipswich Connection. Kevin is the weakness . . . he's overrated and the other two run around trying to make him look good.' He came to Glenn Lazarus. 'Big, fat and slow, provides ordinary go-forward.' One of our blokes was down as a 'thug'. Another was 'soft'. As Wayne read on, we were torn between rage and disbelief. We got pretty damned emotional, and couldn't wait to make St George pay. I was seething. After learning what St George said about me, I thought: 'I'll give it to these bastards.'

It was years before Wayne got around to telling us he'd pulled a swifty and the tip sheet was a fake. He'd made the whole thing up with former Brisbane Norths coach and Broncos match committee member Bob Bax. Bogus tip sheets were a common ploy back in the 1950s when a coach wanted to fire up his men before a big match. But as we boarded the plane for Sydney and our return bout with Saints, we didn't know we'd been conned, and we were spewing.

There was plenty of needle in the 1993 grand final. A number of things were motivating us to wallop our old Dragon rivals. In a bad-tempered final premiership-round match, in front of 58,593 fans at ANZ Stadium, St George beat us 16–10. Their tactics were to slow the game down; they feigned injury and lay all over us when we were trying to play the ball quickly. The loss hit us hard. It gave Saints a psychological edge, because they'd repelled the best attack we could throw at them for long periods at a time in their two-tries-to-one win. And even worse, our defeat put us in the life-or-death situation of contesting the finals from fifth spot. One loss and we were out.

First up, we met Manly in the minor preliminary semi. A win to us, 36–10. Our attack clicked, and I was content with how I played. The following week we played Canberra and in a lightning-quick match we came out on top 30–12. As usual, it was great to go well against Laurie. Canterbury was next in the preliminary final, and Kerrod starred in our tough 23–16 win. Gee, looking back to that era, there were so many wonderful five-eighths going around. In our three finals appearances to date, I'd found myself opposed to Cliff Lyons, Laurie Daley and Terry Lamb, every one an all-time great of the game.

As grand final day approached, Saints coach Brian Smith went on the radio and said his team were pleased to be playing us in the premiership decider. 'I'm certainly glad we're getting a shot at them, because they're not good at handing out accolades. If they hadn't got there they would have told the world, "*We* didn't get there, so you haven't beaten the best."' Then came even more drama – and motivation. At the grand final breakfast attended by both sides at a Sydney hotel, Smith was handed the microphone and was asked to tell the audience why he believed Saints would win the big one. He declared that St George would be premiers because they were a better team and he was a better coach. In the cold light of hindsight, he obviously meant to say that Saints had *improved* since we beat them in the 1992 grand final, and that with that experience and another season's coaching under his belt he was an *improved* coach. But so high were feelings running in those electric last days that a number of Broncos chose to interpret Smith's words as meaning that Saints were *better* players than Brisbane, and that he was a *better* coach than Wayne. Saints, for their part, were making much of a newspaper column written by Glenn Lazarus, in which he said he didn't rate them as a premiership threat. Lazzo later changed his tune – but such incidents were petrol poured onto an already raging fire.

We burst onto the Sydney Football Stadium that Sunday, 26 September 1993, champing at the bit. Tina Turner's pre-game performance – mimed, I found out later – was still ringing in our ears as Greg McCallum blew kickoff. From the start we could see that Saints were right off their game. They couldn't seem to regroup after they lost their gun prop Jason Stevens with a shocking hand injury in the first minute. They made many uncharacteristic unforced errors. David Barnhill lost the ball three times, Noel Goldthorpe kicked out on the full, usually safe Ricky Walford dropped an easy catch. Right on the 20-minute mark, Saints' prop Tony Priddle forced a pass and the ball went loose, I recovered, broke into the clear and when I came to the last line of defence I passed to Chris Johns who darted over for a try. Nine minutes later I passed inside into a gap, Terry Matterson ran on to the ball full-pelt and scored. We controlled the game from then on, and wrapped it up 12 minutes from fulltime when Julian O'Neill ran a Saints kick strongly back into play and Mark Hohn, Kerrod, Alf, Alan Cann and Andrew Gee combined to send Willie Carne over in the corner. At the end, it was 14–6, three tries to nil.

Compared to the exhilarating razzle-dazzle of the 1992 grand final with all its breathtakingly spectacular moments, 1993 was a lacklustre affair, though a sweet and satisfying victory nonetheless. Winning in 1993 was harder than in 1992 because as premiers we were the team all the other sides wanted to beat when they played us, so they lifted their game. Also, I reckon the playing standard was higher in 1993. And, of course, we'd had to win the grand final from fifth spot. To do so we'd had to beat four class acts in Manly, Canberra, Canterbury and St George in a gruelling, sudden death series of games. Wayne was so proud of us. 'What people forget is the hard, cold fact that we are a team,' he said after the grand final. 'And the past few matches showed what a fine team we are, not just a gathering of individual stars.'

Tina Turner joined us in the post-match celebrations on the field. Of course, she made a bee-line for me, the best-looking Bronco. What was a fella to do? I put my arm around the superstar as we belted out our club song. I felt so good. I'd had a strong game, setting up two of our three tries, and Kerrod played a blinder. In one of his finest performances he toiled all day, tackling his heart out, and his dummy half play was superb. And after all that, he still had it in him to break clear and play his part in Willie's try. David Middleton, writing in *Rugby League 1994*, the NSWRL's official yearbook, noted: 'There were few standouts in a solid team performance by the Broncos, but the Walters brothers, Kevin and Kerrod, were probably the pick. The pair each played a part in two of the three tries scored. And second rower Trevor Gillmeister completed his three-year career with the Broncos on the perfect note. His defence throughout the finals series was of the highest order.'

As the shadows lengthened over the Sydney Football Stadium after the grand final, Alf bounced around in that stylish beer-can hat he'd worn the same time the previous year. Another memorable moment was the triumphant but sad expression on Gilly's face as he held the Winfield Cup trophy high above his head after playing his last match in the Broncos colours. Terry Matterson said of his close mate, a victim of the salary cap: 'You've got to give it to Gilly after what's happened. He never dropped his bundle and really dug in for the players. He's a great bloke and a great player and it's going to be very difficult replacing him. We're all going to miss him. He's a champion.'

Chris Johns and I had an extra reason to celebrate. Look at the match video today, and at the end of the game, you'll see an unusually wide smile on Chris's face. The reason was that, after our loss to Saints in the last premiership-round game, he placed a bet of $5000 at 4–1 with a certain Brisbane bookie that we'd win the grand final. The bookie snapped it up, because we sure had the job ahead of us at that stage. Chris asked me if I wanted a bit of the action and I said: 'Not just yet, mate.' He replied: 'You're crazy! We're gonna win the comp, no worries.' Chris is a super-confident guy, and I recall how he picked us up in that worrying period after the loss to Saints. His refusal to contemplate anything less than a grand final victory inspired us all then, even though he was going through a terrible patch at home when his wife Lisa was diagnosed with a tumour on her acoustic nerve which required major surgery. Thank God, it turned out to be benign. In spite of my friendship with Johnsie, I told him I wasn't interested in the bet.

I'm superstitious about betting on football games, because the only other time I did so was years ago in an Under-18 match and we got flogged. We hadn't been beaten all year and I bet on us to win the grand final and we lost. It wasn't a lot of money, $120 or something. So after lots of thought, I told Chris: 'No.' Then of course we won all our semis and finals and only Saints stood between us and the Winfield Cup. In the dressing room before the grand final he came up to me and said: 'Kevvie, you can still have some of this money – I'll even let you in now. I'll let you in for $500 if you want.' I said: 'Just let me run out onto the field and when I get out there I'll let you know.' We ran out and I got this enormous surge of enthusiasm and knew we were not going to be beaten that day. I went over to Johnsie's wing and said: 'Mate, I'm in.' We shook hands and that was it. I picked up about two grand out of it. Chris won $20,000. Imagine how good we felt when I put him over for our first try.

While the grand final may not have been of as high a standard as 1993's, the celebration party back in Brisbane was. Queenslanders' priorities were set in stone a few days before when Broncos stories and photos – including one about Glenn Lazarus's injured ankle – shoved the announcement that Sydney had won the right to stage the 2000 Olympics off the front pages. Once more, on grand final night the airport was jammed with supporters; one or two may have even been sober. More than 6000 turned up at King George Square to hear Kerrod and me belt out our 1992 Top 10 smash hit, 'Hey, Hey, We're the Broncos'. When the cheers died down, I rubbed it into our opponents. 'Have St George scored yet?' I yelled. Gilly announced that he wanted to have a beer with every single fan. Six thousand beers might have stretched even Gilly's capacity, but over the next few days he made a solid attempt to keep his word. As in 1992, Alfie Langer surfed the crowd.

What Alf did later that night back at the Leagues Club had some southern critics thinking he'd been dropped on his head in the melee. After many beers, he took the microphone and sang at the top of his voice: 'St George can't play! St George can't play!' The equally well-oiled crowd joined in. Then, as Channel 7's and the ABC's cameras rolled, Alf, still on stage, skolled a beer and let out a big burp – it was just Alf being Alf. Next day the footage was screened around Australia and created a furore. 'What sort of image is Langer giving to the game, acting like a lout and being unsportsmanlike about the opposition?' demanded the media commentators. Proud Saints fans were enraged, and Dragons have long memories. They have never forgiven Alf. Every time he appeared at Kogarah the crowd targeted him mercilessly, calling out: 'Alf can't play! Alf can't play!' And not just Alf. They give it to the whole team, and especially to players they regard as traitors. Gorden Tallis was on the bench for Saints in the 1993 grand final, just starting the illustrious career that saw him join us a few years later. Now St George crowds reserve special treatment for Gorden. At Stadium Australia for the double-header that kicked off the 1999 season, he was with swimming champ Hayley Lewis when loud boos and sledging came from a bunch of Saints fans. Gorden turned to Hayley and said: 'Crikey, what've *you* done wrong?!'

I was disappointed in Channel 7 and the ABC for screening the footage of our celebrations. For goodness' sake, no one encourages drunkenness, but it *was* grand final night and if you can't have a drink and be outrageous then, when can you? Also, it was an adults-only function. There were no kids. And while Alf liked nothing more than winning, he always respected his opponents, as any true professional does. Running that footage did Alf's image a lot of damage for a while. Now that he's retired, everyone thinks Alf was always loved by all, but it's a fact that when *Inside Sport* ran an article on the most hated sportsmen of 1993 Alf was on top of the list because of the bad publicity of that grand final night.

But as we celebrated our second successive premiership, all that was tomorrow's problem. At the start of the semis, Alf had got us together and said: 'Look, if we win the comp, we're all getting our heads shaved.' And we did win, so we did. At some stage in the proceedings – like a lot of things that happened that night, it's all a bit of a blur now – Sharon Gee and a couple of the other girls scalped us. Even Wayne got the razor. Did we look ugly! Losing their hair really brought the few good-looking blokes in our team, like Willie Carne and Steve Renouf, down to our level. We partied long into the night. Alf, Kerrod and I kept phoning Saints boss Geoff Carr at the St George Leagues Club, rubbing in our victory. 'Have Saints scored yet?' we were still wanting to know.

CHAPTER SEVEN

# LOSING IT

Grand final day 1994 was a little different to 1992 and 1993. Instead of running onto the Sydney Football Stadium to defend our title, we all gathered around the TV at Alf's place, watching Canberra beat Canterbury 36–12. Alf and Janine Langer turned it on for us, with lamb, pork and beef on the spit and lots to drink. But delicious as the spread was, we all had a bitter taste in our mouth. I joked to *Rugby League Week*'s Tony Durkin: 'When I was a young bloke, I always looked forward to watching the grand final with all my mates. A feed, a few beers, and then into the game. It was always a big day – one of the biggest of the year. This grand final day was really no different to what we did back then. We are all good mates at the Broncos and we had a big day. We enjoyed the social outing. Not as good as grand final day last year, mind you, or the year before.'

I was jealous when I saw the Raiders and Bulldogs

players at the grand final breakfast on TV. 'Seeing all the guys there really brought it home to me. Suddenly it hit me – the biggest day of the year and I won't be there. It was an awful feeling. I felt sick in the stomach, and pretty useless. But at least we know who is to blame: no one but ourselves. We took the toughest possible route to the grand final, as we did last year, but this time we dipped out. You have to want to win every week, not just when you need to. One day you dig in the well, and there's nothing there. That's just what happened to us in our sudden death elimination semi against Norths when we went down 15–14.'

That grand final night, as celebrations raged in the national capital, Brisbane was dead quiet, the airport and King George Square deserted, the crime rate back to normal.

'This may be a good lesson for us,' Kerrod reflected at season's end. 'You can't win games on brilliance alone. You have to work for victories. We just weren't mentally prepared throughout the year. Our minds weren't on the job.'

We didn't deserve to retain our title. Individually, we played OK, good enough for Wendell Sailor, Michael Hancock, Glenn Lazarus, Steve Renouf, Alf and me to make the 1994 Kangaroo tour of England and France. But somehow, as a team, the wheels fell off. We lost our hunger to win in 1994. Wayne said towards the end of the season: 'They have lost the sting in their tail. There is a distinct lack of motivation out there and I'm at a loss to work out why. There has been a lot of talk about what they are going to do, but not much action. This bunch of players have been to the top of the mountain, and are seemingly not all that keen about going back there . . . We've lost the plot.'

We started the season badly, drawing with Parramatta and losing to the Gold Coast and, sweet revenge for them, St George. We were inconsistent all year. Two wins would be followed by a loss until the second half of the second round of the premiership when we won six out of seven. That got us into the semis in fourth spot. We beat Manly 16–4 after I put Steve Renouf into space and he scored an 80-metre try against the run of play, but we came unstuck against the Bears. They beat us 15–14 and that was the end of us for the year. At the final siren Alf bitterly hurled his mouthguard away. The Broncos' dreams of an extended premiership run, like the great Saints sides of the 1950s and 1960s, had turned to dust. An added downer was that we also lost our World Club Champions title to a fired-up Wigan, who beat us 20–14 at ANZ in front of a crowd of 54,000.

There were reasons for our failures. Perhaps we were complacent after winning two grand finals in a row. 'We got too comfortable in our success,' said Wayne. 'It's the same as anyone in life who has success. You sit back and wait for someone to do something. If the boys were perfect, I'd be out of a job. I'd have more hair and I'd smile a lot more.' We had a wicked injury toll. A crook knee kept Paul Hauff out almost all season. Willie Carne was badly battered by a series of head knocks. Lazzo's knee injury saw him play just 14 matches all year. We were bashed up by the judiciary, too. We had five blokes suspended that season, more than any other club. Gavin Allen copped eight matches for elbowing Cronulla's Paul Green in the head. Alan Cann got four weeks for a high tackle. Peter Ryan was outed for three weeks for biting Parramatta's Jason Bell. Steve Renouf was given two weeks for a spear tackle. Kerrod got a fortnight for what the judiciary decided was a spear tackle on Canberra forward David Furner. Alf got cited along with Kerrod for the tackle, on Furner, but Alf was exonerated. Not one of our guys had been sent off. In each case the referee deemed a penalty sufficient punishment. Each bloke was cited after the game. When Kerrod was suspended, he lashed out. He accused the NSWRL judiciary of discriminating against the Broncos, and Wayne and our chief executive John Ribot backed him to the hilt and said the Broncos were being victimised. 'I like to think we play within the rules,' said Wayne. 'I'm filthy at players who concede penalties.'

The NSWRL demanded to know why Kerrod shouldn't be fined $10,000 for bringing the game into disrepute. He ended up being fined $5000 and he paid out of his own pocket. My brother was unrepentant then and remains unrepentant to this day. 'The ARL decided they were going to get one of us and they knew if they found us both guilty there'd be an uproar, and if they got Alf there'd be an uproar, so that left me. I got hauled up to the judiciary three times and got dudded three times. I'd had enough.'

We were squabbling with the NSWRL all year, and that didn't help our state of mind. We really felt it was us against them.

The crowded rep season didn't help the Broncos' cause because, as usual, the Queensland side was largely made up of Brisbane blokes – Julian O'Neill, Michael Hancock, Steve Renouf, Willie Carne, Alf and me, Andrew Gee and Mark Hohn. And Alf, Michael, Steve and Mark made the Australian team for the one-off 58–0 Test rout of France at Parramatta Stadium. For the first time in my career, I was first choice five-eighth in all three Origin games.

Origin I, the first to be played under the 10-metre ruck rule, ranks with the all-time great rugby league thrillers. With time running out fast we were down 12–4, after Harragon and Mackay had scored tries for them and O'Neill one for us. The game, a titanic struggle with ferocious forward clashes and wide-open running in the backs, was just about out of our grasp. Our coach Wally Lewis was slumped in his seat in the stands. The commentators and most of the crowd had given up on us. But we didn't lie down. With four minutes to go, Alf made a break. From the play the ball it went to Carne, to me, to Renouf, to Mark Coyne who flung a desperation pass. The ball deflected from the arm of our prop Darren Fritz right into the hands of Willie Carne who scored. Meninga converted: NSW 12 – Queensland 10. With 60 seconds left on the clock, the Blues were desperately trying to close down the game. They failed. From deep in our territory, Alf threw a long ball to me standing wide on the left of the ruck. I passed to Carne who shot it out Renouf who accelerated as if fuel-injected. Renouf gave it to Hancock who somehow sent to Darren Smith just as Ettingshausen drove him into the ground. On now to Alf, to Meninga, then to Coyne, who beat Stuart and Fittler and plunged over for the matchwinning try. 'That's not a try. That's a miracle!' Channel 9 caller Ray Warren screamed as Coyne scrambled over and plonked the ball down. We went mad on the field. An unbelievable and unforgettable escape. A delirious Wally hugged everyone he could reach.

The second match of the series was played at the Melbourne Cricket Ground in front of 87,161 people, an Australian record until the 110,000 or so who turned up for the double header at Stadium Australia that kicked off the 1999 season. The Blues shut us out, 14–0. Harragon and Lazzo belted us up front in a dour match. The decider was set for Lang Park. Origin III was extra special because it would be Mal Meninga's last match for Queensland. The Blues were farewelling Benny Elias. The hometown crowd had worked hard on their banners. One read: 'Goodbye Mal. Good riddance Benny!' But we tried too hard to send Mal out a winner and we fumbled and faltered. Crowd villain Elias had the last laugh when he inspired New South Wales to an easy and anticlimactic 29–12 victory. They ran away from us early, largely thanks to two intercept tries, the first when Alf threw the ball to Elias who sent Clyde over, and the second when Brett Mullins intercepted a squeezed pass from Renouf to Carne. It was 18–0 before we got our act together. Gee and Renouf crossed and Mal was trampling the Blues backs. Then again the tide turned and Brad Fittler kicked a field goal that took the wind out of our sails, then he rubbed it in with a try. I did Mal no favours when I hurled a wild pass in his direction with seconds to go. He stretched but couldn't pull it in. The mighty Mal deserved better.

What a rollercoaster year. If there was one game that summed up my mixed fortunes in 1994 it was when we played Canterbury at ANZ in February. I set up tries for Steve Renouf and Chris Johns and scored one myself and I was walking on air, already counting my player of the match booty, but with seconds to go and the Bulldogs trailing only by 6, I came down to earth with a thud. I chipped right into the arms of my old Ipswich Grammar schoolmate Craig Polla-Mounter who ran 80 metres to score. Bulldogs two points down and the deadly Daryl Halligan going for the conversion that would tie the game. My heart was in my boots as he lined up the kick, moved in, connected . . . and missed. Whew! A win to us, 16–14, and I had a new nickname: 'Chipsy', courtesy of Alf.

That year I did another of those question-and-answer sessions with a journo, and some of my answers give a good take on where my life was back then. It was only five years ago, but it seems a lifetime. In those days I drove a Hyundai Sonata. My favourite other team was the Aussie cricket side, my favourite record was Cold Chisel's 'Khe Sanh' (just pipping 'Hey, Hey, We're The Broncos' by that other classic band, The Ipswich Connection). My preferred relaxation was playing with our sons Billy and Jack. Big Macs were my favourite fast food. Laurie and

Cliff Lyons were my toughest opponents. My family and Wayne Bennett had the biggest influence on me. If I won Lotto I was going to put a deposit on a tropical island. If I could be any other sportsman, I'd be Andre Agassi because I fancied myself at tennis and I'd like all his money and to be able to travel the world. If I could relive one moment, what would it be? To be there again at the birth of our children.

It was a blast to be picked a second time to tour with the Kangaroos. Not too many blokes get two trips. This time Kerrod missed out and Steve made the squad, which was skippered by Mal. I enjoyed the tour. I couldn't unseat Laurie as first-choice five-eighth, but I knuckled down and played nine games, against the Great Britain Under-21 side, the Wales and Cumbria rep teams, the English club sides Castleford, Sheffield, St Helens and Warrington, as well as the French President's XIII and France B. I captained Australia against St Helens. We won 32–14 and I had a running battle with referee Colin Morris. Things came to a head when coach Bob Fulton sent word onto the field that Morris had given us two sets of four tackles instead of six. I fronted him and accused him of shortchanging us. 'Excuse me, sir,' I said, 'but you've just given us two sets of four tackles.' He said: 'I don't think so.' I said: 'I'm pretty sure you did.' He yelled: 'Keep that up, son, and I'll put you in the bin.' By now I was enjoying myself and there was no way I was going to back down. At last, Morris said: 'That's it! Ten minutes in the bin!' I copped it.

As I ran off the field, the St Helens crowd was

singing: 'Dirty Aussie bastard! Dirty Aussie bastard!' I loved it. In fact, I love playing in England with the stands right up close to the field. The atmosphere is electric. It's a great shame that Kangaroo tours are a thing of the past now. Young kids in our game are missing out on a lot. I know I learned a lot about footy and life on those trips to England and France. I was happy with my form in 1994 and enjoyed the footy and the tour. Just like the 1990 'Roos, we lost only one game, and as in 1990, that was the First Test against Great Britain at Wembley. But we won the next two Tests convincingly at Old Trafford and Leeds to retain the Ashes. Just one Test in France and that finished with a 74–0 thrashing for the locals.

I missed Kim, Jack and Billy desperately. I was always on the phone to home, begging and pleading with Kimmie to come to England and bring the boys. Taking two toddlers on that 25-hour flight could not have been a picnic, but Kim and the boys came and it was terrific. I'd planned to spend the off-season with the London Broncos, but by the end of the tour I'd had enough of being away from home and so turned them down. They were pretty disappointed, and it would have been a great experience for me and the family, but instead we returned to Brissie for Christmas with our family and preparation for season 1995. The Broncos were determined to put the disappointments of 1994 behind them and roar back with premiership No. 3.

As it turned out, 1995 would be a memorable year, but not for football. The Broncos were the catalyst for

Super League, no risk. Looking back, I can see how a lot of league fans saw the Broncos as whingers and trouble-makers. Our management certainly knew how to stirup the establishment and get fans off side. Super League sprang from our endless bitter squabbling with the New South Wales Rugby League, which ran the Winfield Cup. We believed John Quayle and his team had not given us a fair go. We believed they resented our management running the Broncos as an entrepreneurial profit-making business. We believed the League was trying to bring us back to the field. So we took our concept for revolutionising the game and the way it was run to Rupert Murdoch and News Ltd. The rest is history.

No, in 1995 football became a sideshow. The year will be remembered forever for the Super League war, for broken friendships and media moguls and huge player payments. On one side were the clubs that stayed with the establishment – Manly, Sydney City, St George, Illawarra, Newcastle, Norths, Gold Coast, South Queensland, South Sydney, the Tigers, Wests and Parramatta. Aligned with Super League were the Broncos, Cronulla, Penrith, the Bulldogs, Canberra, Auckland, North Queensland and the Western Reds. It was the year Australian rugby league tore itself apart.

CHAPTER EIGHT

# LAUGHING AT LIFE

The Super League war affected me as much as anyone. It has been well documented in a number of books and newspaper features, so I'm not going to go into the nitty-gritty here. Alf's book gives a good account from the Broncos' bunker, so check it out in *Alf: The Allan Langer Story*. (Alf, you know where to send the royalties, mate!) Also, I decided when I sat down to write my story that I didn't want to do a controversial book, giving sensational revelations about the private lives of famous rugby league stars. Sure, there are blokes in our game who I wouldn't invite around for dinner. I have my loves and hates about rugby league and the blokes who play and run it and commentate on it, but it's never been my go to bag people in public and I'm not going to start now. I'm known as a bit of a clown, and that suits me, because if we didn't have a laugh we would all go insane. I'd rather remember the fun stuff.

Like the time Kerrod, Alf and I became pop stars. Just before the 1992 grand final, we recorded 'Hey, Hey, We're the Broncos'. It was a gimmick, a bit of a joke, cooked up by Kerrod and our manager Barry Collins. We had no idea it would became a national hit. I know I said before that the Monkees stole the words and tune from us, but I'll confess now that it was the other way around. We changed their lyrics, and a music track was recorded. Then, calling ourselves The Ipswich Connection, Kerrod, Alf and I went to the Sony recording studio and sang the new words over the music. It took us three takes, and even though we can't hold a tune to save our lives, the technical wizards did their work, and the stupid bloody thing sounded half-OK. It sold more than 7000 copies and made No. 1 in the Queensland charts and No. 28 nationally.

It took off because the timing was perfect. There was all the excitement and hype because it was our first grand final, and then we won it. Unbelievable, and the record rode on the back of that unbelievable atmosphere. There was a lot of money generated from the song, but somehow it didn't find its way into our pockets. Welcome to the music industry. Once we were on tour in a coach and the ABC rock video show 'Rage' was on the TV and on came 'Hey, Hey, We're the Broncos'. It was wild, bloody hilarious. The other Broncos had been bagging Kerrod, Alf and me about being big-time rock stars, and suddenly we're on 'Rage'. I've still got a copy of the record at home and the kids play it. At training just the other day we were in the dressing room and someone put the track on the sound system. I'm thinking what bloody idiots we were to do it, then I thought: 'Hey, that sounds all right . . .' Unfortunately, for all its success, there were no million dollar offers to record a follow-up. Wonder why not?

One night The Ipswich Connection nearly joined fellow chart-toppers Elvis, John Lennon and Michael Hutchence in Rock'n'Roll Heaven. And I blame Ricky Stuart. Over the years I learned plenty watching Ricky play. For Canberra, NSW and Australia, and now Canterbury, the bloke has been one of the true champions of league. But not everything he's taught me has been about football. He had this totally stupid and dangerous trick of covering the eyes of cabbies when they were driving. I'd been with Ricky a few times when he'd done it and it was a scream to see how the poor driver would react, so once on our way home after a good liquid night out, Alf and Kerrod and I were in a cab and I thought: 'I'll give this a go myself!' I was sitting directly behind the driver and I covered his eyes with my hands. He was on the straight and didn't seem too worried. So a little later I tried it again. I put my hands over his eyes. But this time he lost it completely. He screamed to a stop and swung around and grabbed me and yelled: 'Listen here, you smart arse, I don't mind you covering my eyes on the straight – but *don't* blind me when I'm goin' around corners!'

Ernest was a racehorse. Back in 1986, when Kim and I were trying to raise some money to go to live in Canberra where I'd signed for the Raiders, we had about $500 to our name and were trying to increase our bank balance. I was struggling to make ends meet on my apprentice carpenter's wage. So Kim's dad Buddy persuaded me to become his partner in a horse. One weekend, just before we headed south, Ernest was racing in Caloundra and Kim and I went for broke. We bet the lot, $500, on him. Near the end of the race, Ernest was doing well and was a real chance to win. We were screaming and yelling with joy. Then the jockey dropped his whip. Ernest faded and finished unplaced. I was almost in tears. I wanted to fight the jockey but lucky for him he was smart enough to make himself scarce. Driving home in a fury I was booked for speeding and fined $130. Not a good day. But not bad enough to cure me of the horses. Over the years I've been a partner in a few nags and none have done too well. Old Ernest turned out to be the best of the lot. He won three starts out of 12, including wins at Bundamba and Gatton. I've always found racehorses are fun but, gee, they eat holes in your pocket.

Alf is a more committed racetrack punter than me, but he'll bet on anything. We always had a $100 bet at the beginning of each new season over who would score most tries in the year. Every try I scored brought a smart-arse remark from Alf, and I'd gee him up when he crossed the line. I lost the bet most years, but I never settled. Alf once bet Glenn Lazarus and me that he could stay off the punt longer than we could stay away from cigarettes. I broke first. We'd just played a game and I was relaxing and enjoying a few beers and I lit up. I thought Alf was nowhere around, but no such luck. The bloke's got antennae when there's money to be won, and he sprung me. I had no choice but to cough up. You guessed it, Alf took my money and went straight out and put it on a horse – and it won.

I'm not a big racetrack punter, but I do like going to the casino and playing blackjack. I'm capable of going a little bit silly at the tables. The atmosphere gets to me. We all used to go to Jupiters on the Gold Coast, but that came to a halt after Julian O'Neill had a few well-publicised nights there. Suddenly we weren't so welcome. Most of the capital cities have casinos these days, and we've been known to front when we're in town. In Auckland during the Super League Tri-Series between Queensland, NSW and New Zealand in 1997, the Maroons were in Auckland and a few of us went to the casino. Knowing how money can run through my fingers at a casino, I thought I'd be clever and only take $200 along. I left the rest of my money in my room. I blew that $200 quick-smart but wasn't too downhearted because I knew most of my money was safely back in my hotel room. Darren Lockyer, my room-mate on the tour, was with me, and he did his dough too. Suddenly he disappeared, but returned a short time later and grinned: 'We're right, mate! We've got more funds!' I said: 'What do you mean?' He said: 'Oh, I went back to our room and got all my

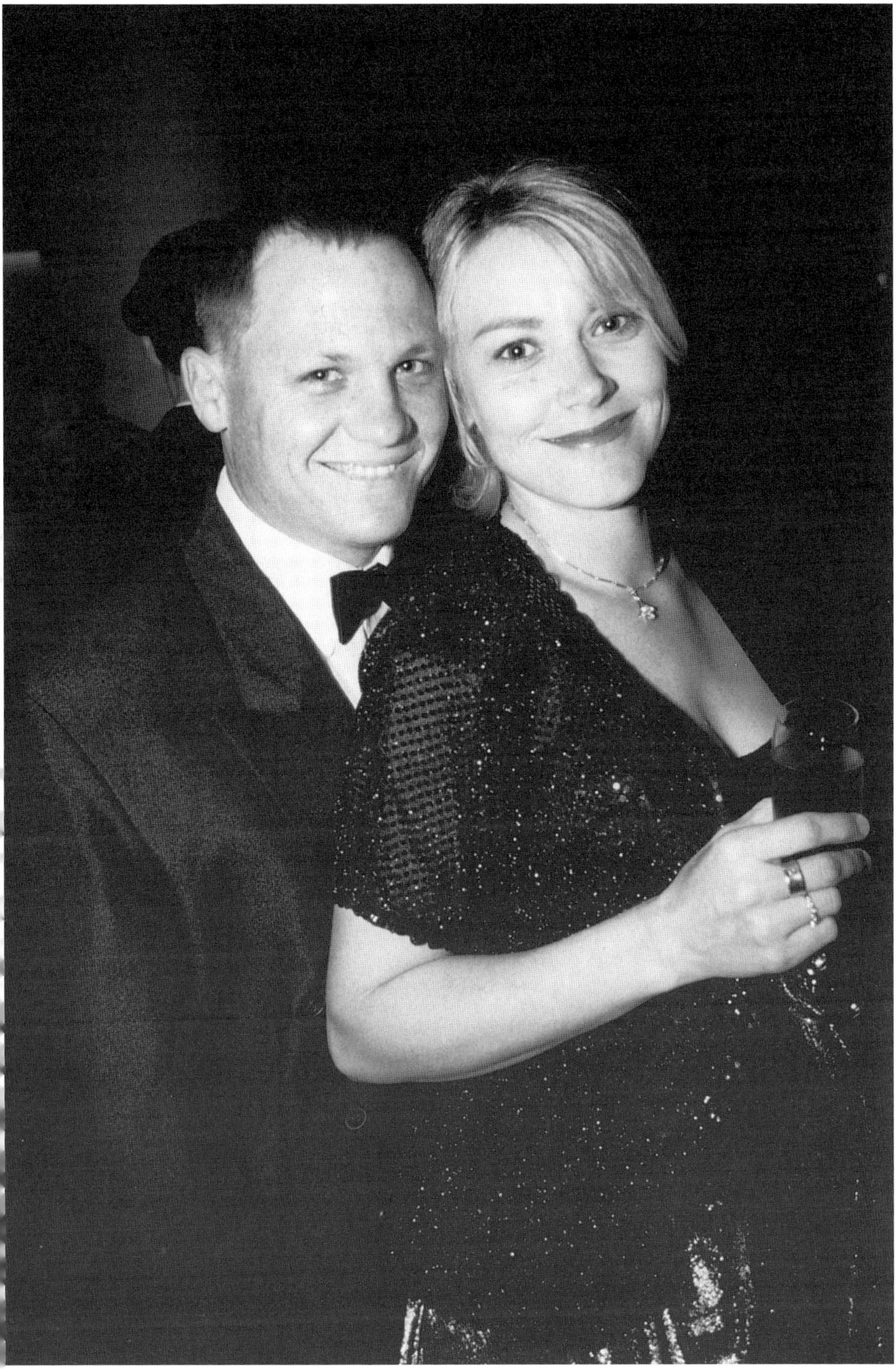

Kim, seven months pregnant with Jett, was radiant at the 1996 Broncos Presentation Ball. Her brave smile belies her illness. Jett was born two weeks later, and then her chemotherapy began.

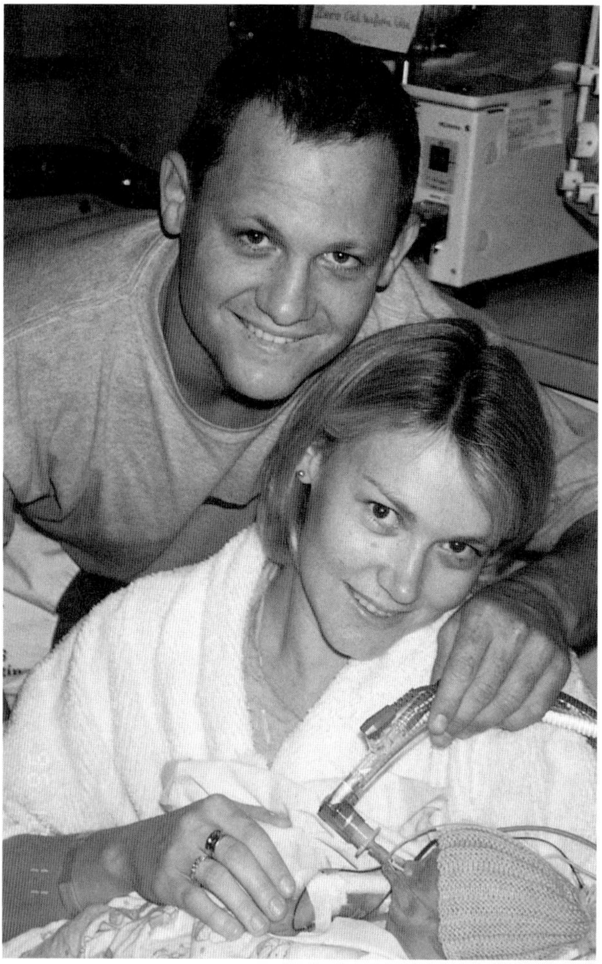

Jett, a couple of weeks old at Brisbane's Mater Hospital, with his doting mum and dad.

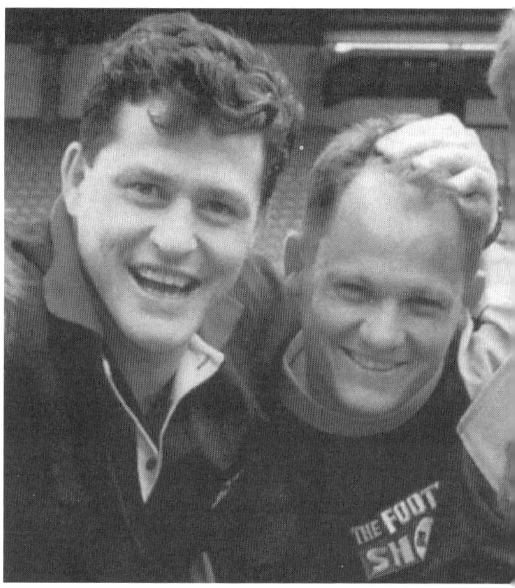


You've got to laugh. This is me in 1996 with my mate, the irrepressible, talented – and tragic – Peter Jackson. We were hamming it up for a 'Footy Show' photo. (Photo courtesy of *Gold Coast Bulletin*)

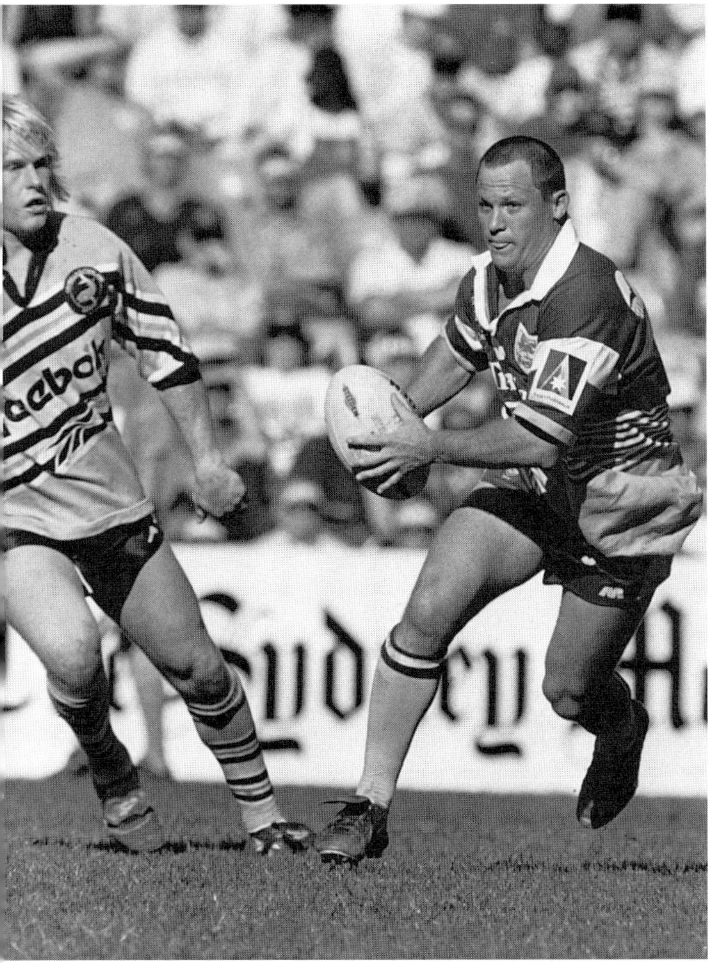

Scheming against Cronulla in a 1996 semi-final. To no avail, because we were beaten by the Sharks and knocked out of the premiership race. That's Nathan Long about to pounce.

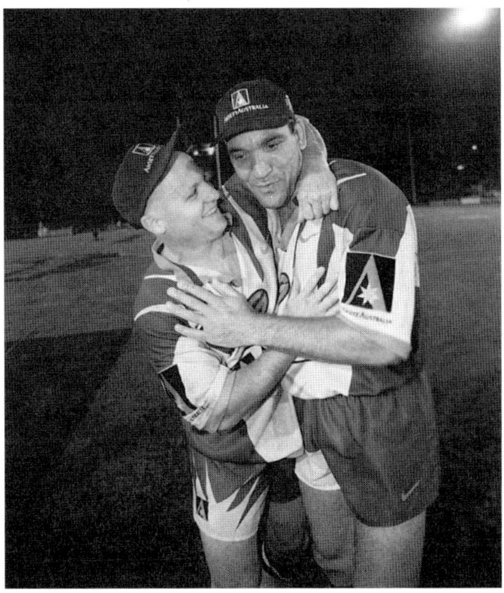

I celebrate with the ferocious Gorden Tallis after the Broncos whipped Cronulla in the 1997 Super League grand final. Gorden, one of the hardest men in the game, is a good man to have on your side in a crisis.

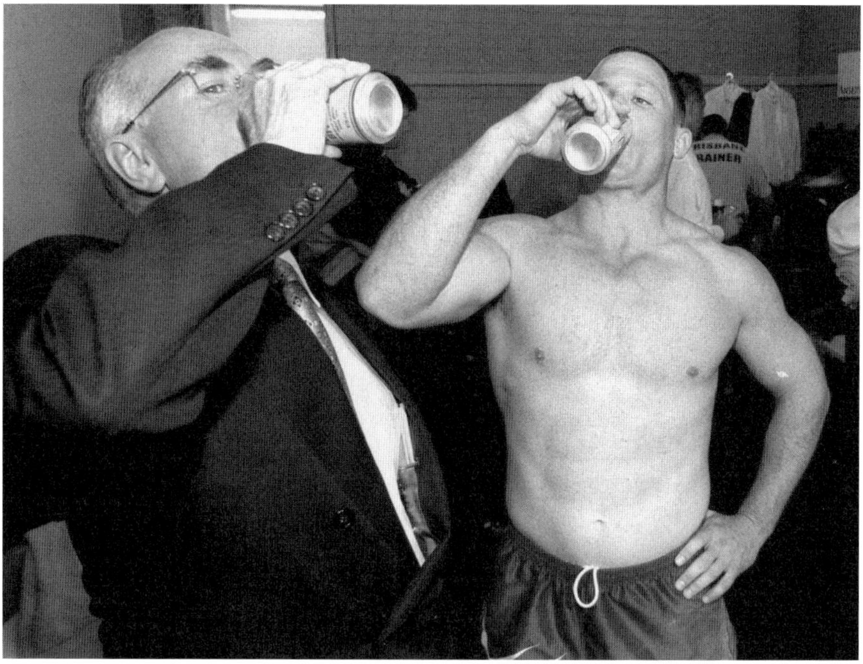

There's Kevin Walters, but who's the bloke in the suit? Just joking, Mr Howard. The Prime Minister joined our dressing room celebration after we beat the Canterbury Bulldogs in the 1998 grand final. (Photo courtesy of News Ltd.)

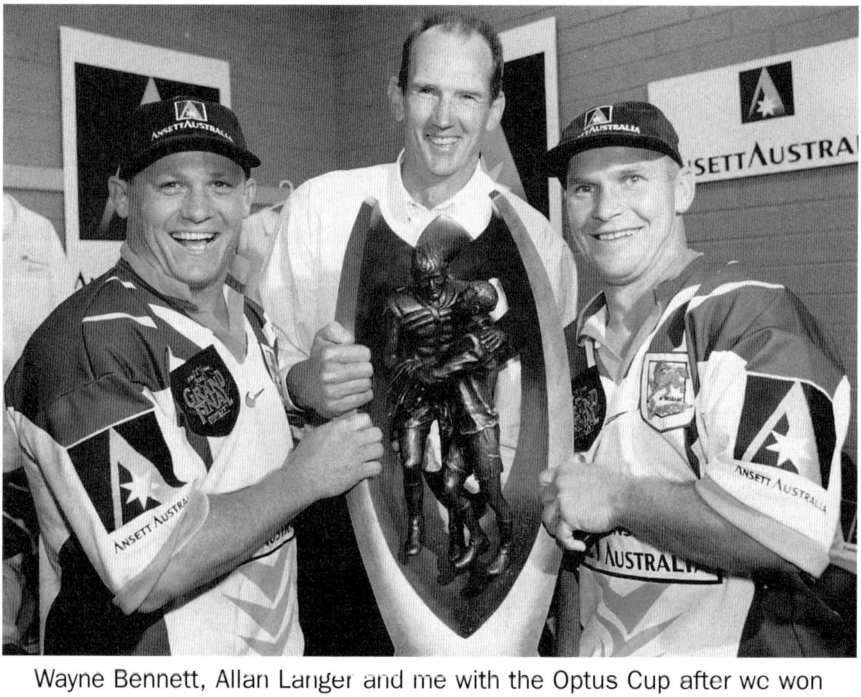


Wayne Bennett, Allan Langer and me with the Optus Cup after we won the 1998 grand final. (Photo courtesy of David Kapernick, Queensland Newspapers)

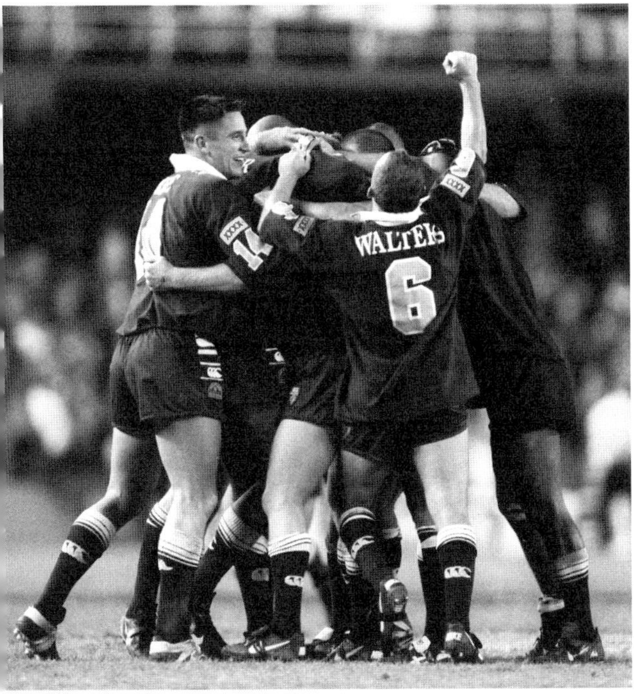


'This one's for you, Kim!' I salute the heavens as we pull off a miracle last-minute win in the 1998 State of Origin I, at Sydney Football Stadium. Steve Price looks on. (Photo courtesy of Action Photographics)

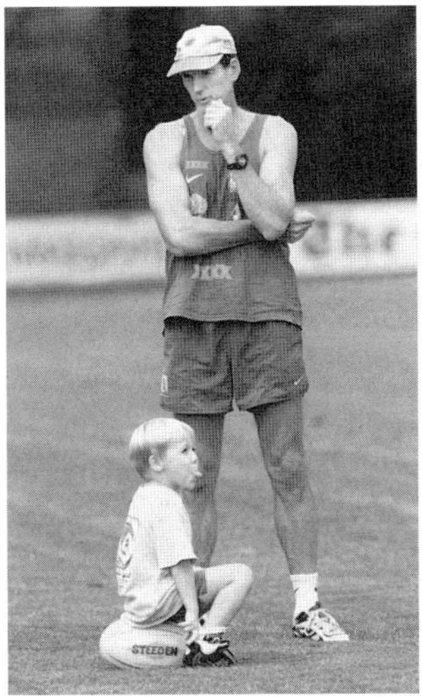

My boy Billy shows what he thinks of master coach Wayne Bennett's tactics at Broncos training in '99. Actually, he's poking his tongue out at Gorden Tallis. Bad move either way. (Photo courtesy of David Kapernick, Queensland Newspapers)

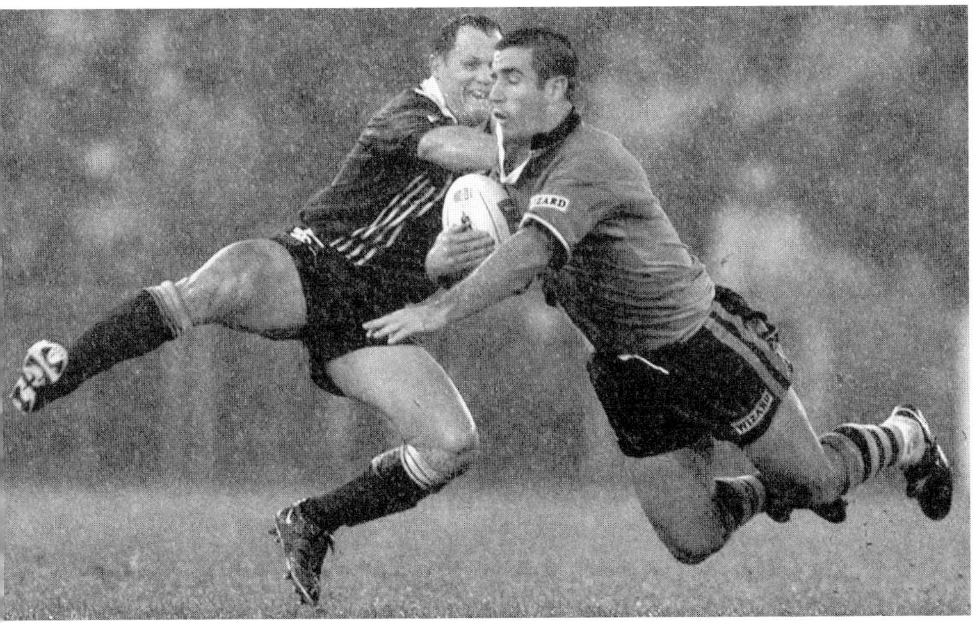

It was a case of 'take your partner' as Andrew Johns and I narrowly avoided a collision in State of Origin II, 1999, at Stadium Australia. I skippered the Maroons in our 12–8 loss. (Photo courtesy of Reuters Australia)

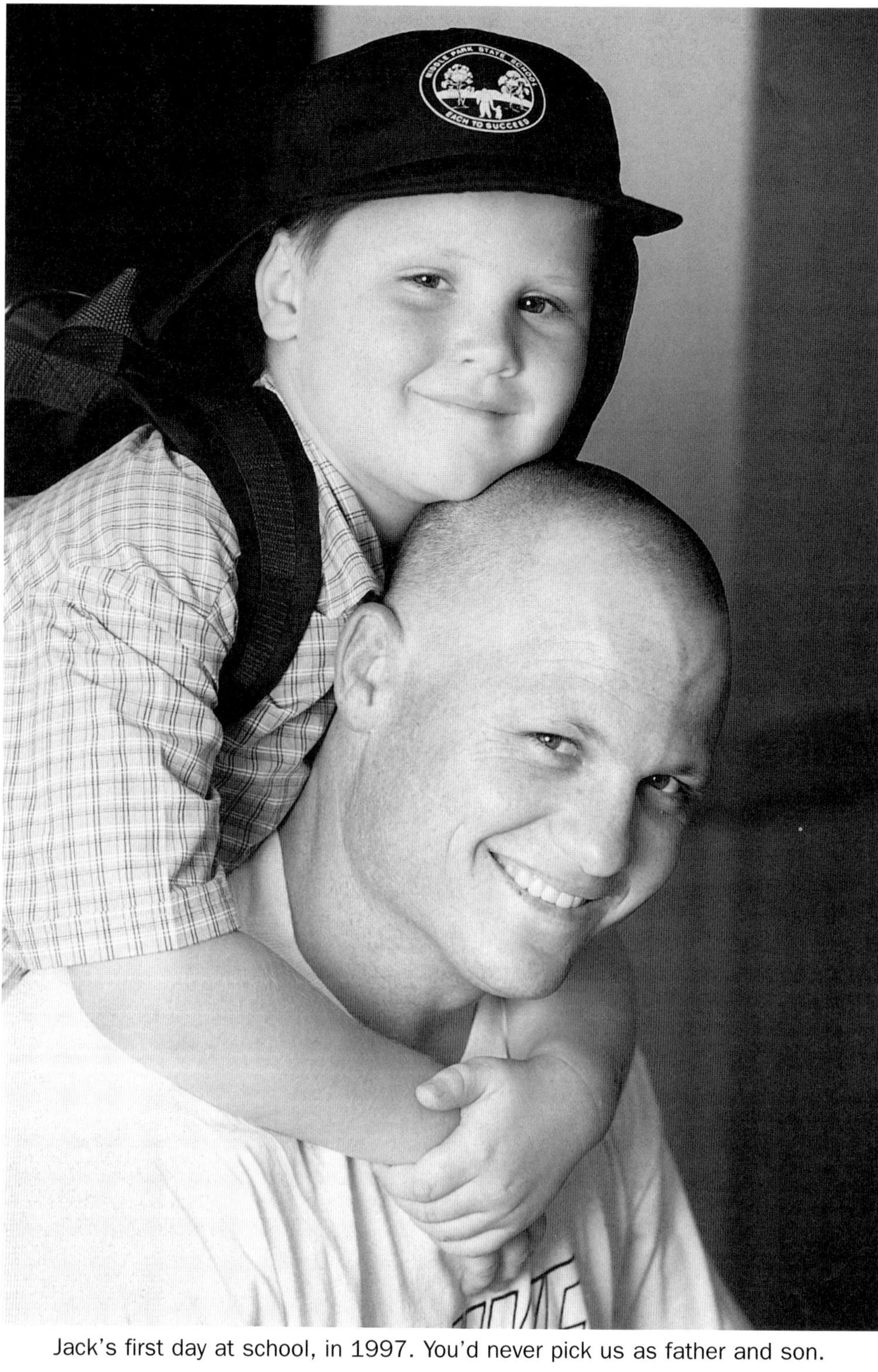

Jack's first day at school, in 1997. You'd never pick us as father and son.

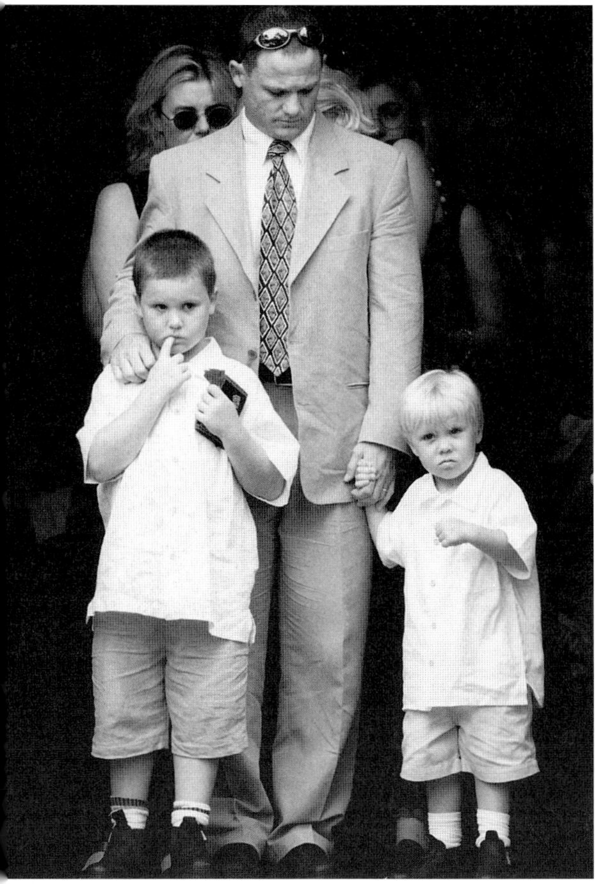

The worst of times: Jack, Billy and me at Kim's funeral, February 1998. (Photo courtesy of the *Courier-Mail*)

Kim would be so pleased to know the breast cancer counselling service in her name has helped many fellow sufferers. With Wesley Breast Clinic director Dr Cherrell Hirst, I spoke at a Kim Walters Choices Program function in 1998. (Photo courtesy of the *Courier-Mail*)

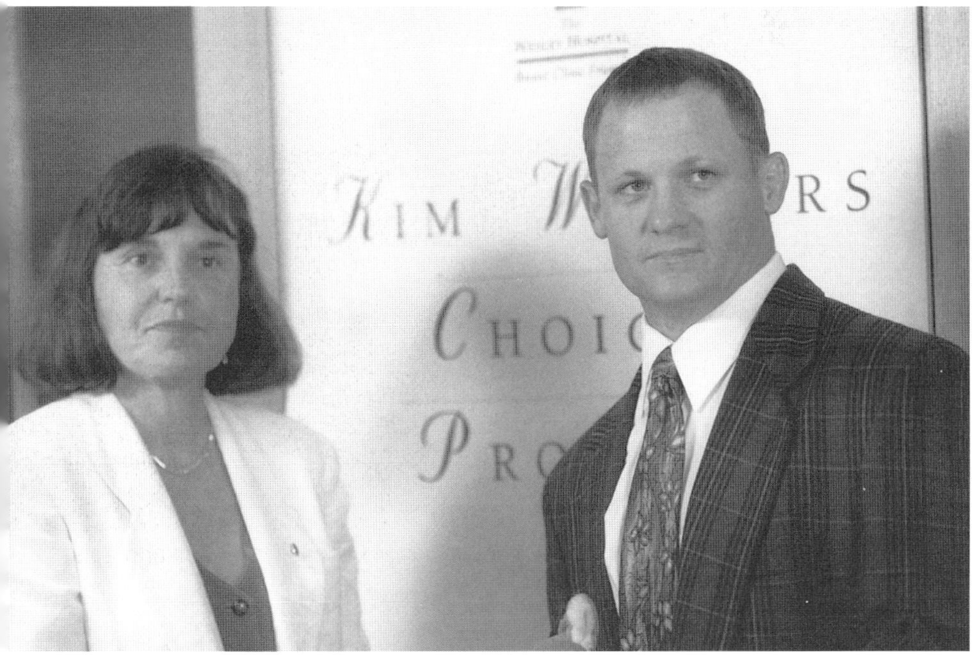

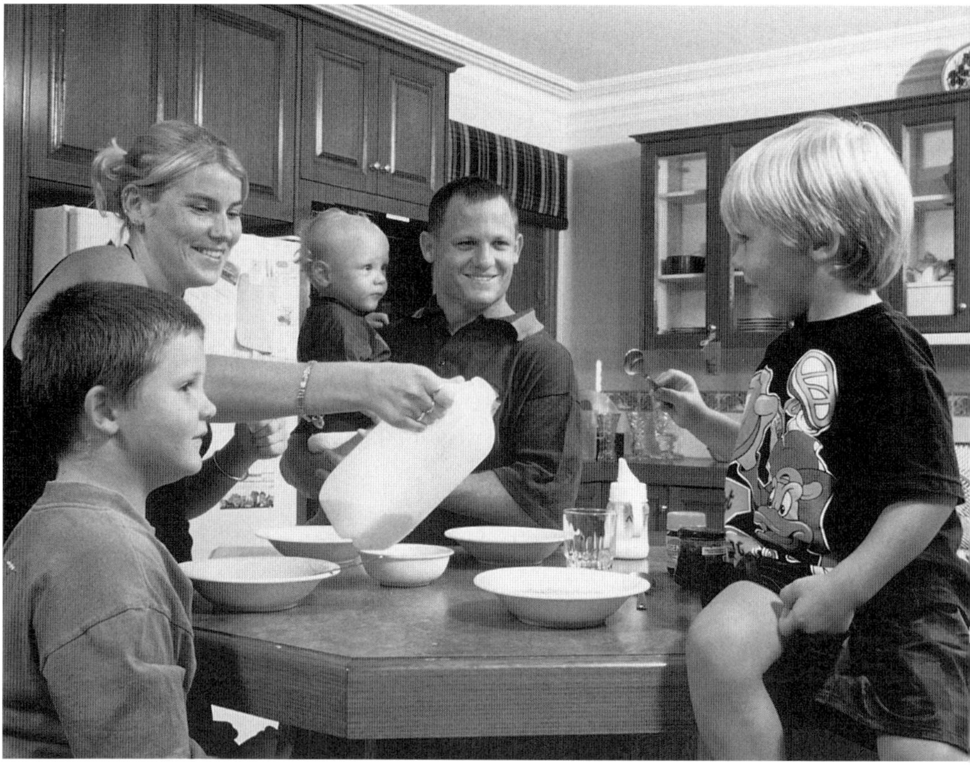

Breakfast chaos in the Walters household, 1998, as Kim's sister Kelly makes sure Jack, Jett, Billy and I get our morning nourishment. I will never be able to thank Kelly enough for her support during Kim's illness.

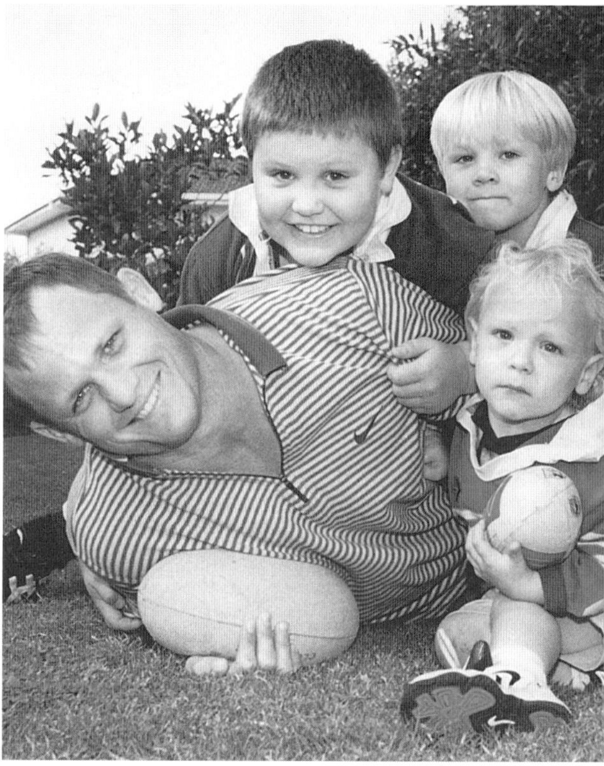

Gang-tackled at home by my boys Jack, Billy and Jett. The two youngest are the spitting image of Kim, while Jack looks like guess who ... (Photo courtesy of David Kapernick, the *Courier-Mail*)

money and all your money and I've just given it to Alf.' As he was speaking, Alf was losing our cash. Every last cent.

I returned to the hotel a shattered man. I'd lost well over a thousand bucks. It was late, so I put off phoning Kim and telling her the terrible news till the next morning. I did not sleep well. I was feeling sick in the guts. Next morning, I bit the bullet and made the call. She wasn't happy. But then she said: 'Now I've got some news for you.' I said: 'Oh, what's that?' She said: 'Billy's driven the car through the garage wall.' I said: 'What!' Kim continued: 'He got into the car to turn the radio on and he knocked the ignition key and the car shot off right through the garage wall. I heard the crash and ran out and the front of the car was sticking right through the bricks.'

Suddenly I forgot all about the lost money. 'Was he hurt?' Thank God he wasn't even scratched. The little Astra was a mess, but that didn't matter either. The scare made me realise how much my family means to me. Nothing else comes close. Kim said that when she stopped shaking she got out the little diary she kept and wrote all about Billy's big adventure so that when he's older he can read all about the day he demolished the garage and the family car. 'This is what you did, son, when you were four . . .'

Kim was never a fan of gambling. She knew it was like a disease that can wreck the lives of the addicted. I like laying a bet on the horses or blackjack, but it's no big deal with me. My favourite flutter is on the football. I love putting a few hundred bucks down on the Friday night TV match and enjoying it with a few friends like Alf Langer and Ben Walker over a couple of beers.

I love appearing on the TV and radio. Cameras and microphones don't scare me, and I admit I'm a bit of a ham. I still appear on 'The Footy Show' from time to time and have a regular radio gig, but for a while there in 1994 my papers were nearly marked 'Never to Appear Live on TV Again'. I was the star of the 'Kevvie Street Beat' segment of 'The Footy Show', and my job was to go out on the streets and into the shopping malls of Brisbane with a Channel 9 camera and sound team and interview ordinary people about rugby league. For some reason I forget now, one day I was carrying a large photograph of John Quayle. Maybe, the NSWRL had been fighting with the Broncos again. Anyway, I walked up to this guy in a shopping plaza and I said: 'Do you know this man?' And he said, 'Yeah, he's an arsehole!' Unfazed, I said: 'Oh, yeah, why's that?' And the bloke let rip about how he thought John Quayle had it in for the Broncos. I didn't think too much about it, just took the film back to Channel 9. I figured they'd cut it and there was no way it'd ever get screened. But no, they ran it on 'The Footy Show' in Queensland and it screened later in New South Wales.

The Sydney switchboard lit up with people complaining, and even the studio audience there booed the segment. Our Brisbane producer John Evans got the sack, and I copped plenty of flak. It was a personal attack, and it ran at a very tense time in

NSWRL–Broncos relations. I think we should all be open to criticism, but calling someone an 'arsehole' is not criticism but a nasty personal attack. Angry John Quayle supporters deluged Channel 9 with letters attacking me. They held me responsible for what the stranger in the shopping mall had said. They said my walking around with the picture of John was asking for trouble. It probably was, too, but I was young and just trying to be funny and it backfired embarrassingly. I regretted it, but I truly meant no harm. People who know me realise it's not part of my makeup to make enemies or hurt people. Personally speaking, I get called an arsehole quite a bit, and it doesn't really worry me too much, but John Quayle was a senior man in rugby league and he wasn't to be messed with.

Then there was the time I appeared on 'Sale of the Century'. Greg Alexander, Billy Moore and I went to Melbourne to compete against stars from other footy codes. It was a lot of fun, and I was disappointed when I got booted out. We made a thousand bucks or so that went to a viewer. It was nice to meet Nicky Buckley, too!

My punchup with Peter Ryan in 1995 made all the papers. It was a serious blue, too, you bet. Peter is a very hard guy, a country boy with bush values who puts steel into the Broncos pack and has helped me with my defence over the years. On the evening in question, I was having a drink at the Paddington Tavern with Peter, Chris Johns (who had a broken arm in plaster at the time) and a few of Peter's mates. When some men drink they get a bit rough and think they're 10-foot tall and bulletproof, and we were all being idiots that night. Peter Ryan started kidney-punching Johnsie and Johnsie kidney-punched him back. It began as a bit of fun, just a bit of playful whacking, but the rumble soon got deadly serious. They were really belting each other. I ran over and said: 'Ryano, you can't do that! He's got a broken arm!' So Peter stopped hitting Johnsie, turned to me and said, 'OK, you'll do, Kevie,' and went *bop!* I hit the deck like a sack of spuds. When my head cleared I jumped up and got stuck into Peter. I was wild. We scuffled all over the place until the fight was broken up. I copped a dusting. The papers said we left the pub as friends and shared a cab home, but that wasn't the case. I was seriously pissed off and as I drove away I gave Peter the finger out the car window. Next day at training everything was OK between us. Just one of the those things between guys, I guess. However, someone at the pub had told the media and it was big news. Kim was disappointed in my behaviour, then her practical side took over and she said: 'Look, if you're going to go around getting into blues you may as well learn how to fight. Go and see Dad and he'll give you some lessons.' I did, but I still haven't put them to use, and I don't intend to. I'm a lover, not a fighter.

Footy players drinking and brawling have made headlines this year, 1999, but apart from these cases I think we all drank more a few years ago before league became truly professional. I know I used to put the beer away a lot more in those wild and carefree days at Canberra and early on at the Broncos than I do now I'm older. It was the done thing then, all the boys got into it. I'd look around at the club or the Paddington Tavern and think: 'Gee, it's all right, I'm not the only one doing this!' Not so much during the week, but after the game I'd flog myself on the grog. It was Kim who made me realise I was not being fair dinkum to myself, not to mention behaving like a goose. Now the footy culture has largely changed, in spite of a few blokes screwing up occasionally, and I'm glad to have changed along with it. I still love a few drinks, but my legless days are behind me.

You don't have to be plastered to have a good time, but it helps if you're a bit crazy. Kim's father Buddy is a bit that way. He's a tough, tough man, a former welterweight amateur boxer (though he's a heavyweight these days!). He's always kept fit and in condition and boasts a gut of iron. He'd let the Broncos give him a whack in the stomach that would double up a normal human being but Buddy wouldn't even flinch. But there is more than one way to skin a father-in-law. I'll let Buddy take up the story: 'I was monkeying around with the Broncos and I was bracing myself and they were punching me in the stomach. Then Wendell Sailor steps up and doesn't hit me once like everyone else, he hits me three times: *whack-whack-whack!* God, it hurt, mainly because I wasn't expecting the second and third blows. I blew up and said to Wendell, "Why'd you hit me three times?" He replied, "Kevvie told me to hit you three times! He told me it'd be OK." Kevin knows I've got a quick temper and loves to torment me. He used to ring me up all the time and change his voice and he'd catch me out every time. When he was touring overseas with the Kangaroos he'd call in the middle of the night and say, "Long distance telephone call from Mr Wong. Will you accept reverse charges?"'

The Broncos accepted Buddy as one of their own. A good move, because he was very effective at settling down the dopes in pubs who always want to have a go at a footballer. A few gentle words from Buddy Facer and they'd make themselves scarce. And Buddy started a Broncos tradition. A few years ago, before we won our first premiership, he made us a promise: 'Win the grand final and I'll burn all the hairs off my chest.' We said: 'You're kidding!' We couldn't believe it. Buddy was as good as his word. In the team bus after we beat Saints we were all playing the fool and some of us were sneaking up behind others and setting fire to their hair with a cigarette lighter. Buddy took this as his cue to keep his promise. He took his shirt off and Alf did the honours with the lighter. The hair sizzled and flamed up and it smelled really bad. 'It doesn't hurt me,' said Buddy. 'I guess I've got a hard old hide.' And he did it every time we won the comp. 'In '98, when we were playing better and better as the semis approached,' recalls Buddy, 'the boys said, "Grow that hair, Buddy, there's gonna be a burn-off".'

Part of the fallout of the Super League bomb that exploded on rugby league in 1995 was the establishment's decision not to select players from clubs aligned with Super League in that year's rep teams. At least in

1995 the Queensland selectors would not be able to use me as a yoyo because I wasn't available for selection in the first place. The club scene progressed as usual. There was talk that Super League clubs would be expelled from the Winfield Cup until Australian Rugby League boss Ken Arthurson said he 'didn't want to punish loyal fans for the actions of irresponsible officials'. At least that meant we Broncos could concentrate on picking up the pieces in the domestic competition. We were all preoccupied by events off the field that season. Our boss John Ribot quit in March to become chief executive of the rebel League, and probably we spent too much time in meetings, like the one in the early Super League days when I stood up and told Ribot that the Broncos players had decided to go with the ARL. When he picked himself up off the floor I assured him I was only joking.

The off-field drama didn't stop us from giving the comp a real shake. Bolstered by the ultra-professional utility star Darren Smith from the Bulldogs, and a wonderful contribution from Wendell Sailor, we came third in the premiership before bad injuries to the world's best centre Steve Renouf (ankle), Alf (quadricep) and Chris Johns (broken arm) and a late loss of form saw us lose both semi-finals – to Canberra and to the Bulldogs, who ended up with the Winfield Cup.

We started the year on fire and won the pre-season Tooheys Challenge and our first seven games straight, including a 36–18 flogging of our old enemies St George at ANZ. Then came a mid-year slump. Canberra caned us 26–0, Manly thumped us 23–4 and

Illawarra belted us 34–18. We regrouped and came out of our slump in the best way – a 60–14 thrashing of Parramatta – then cruised to the semis with a wet sail. Sadly, our exit from the comp was abrupt and decisive. In a classic at ANZ, Canberra were too strong, 14–8. Between us, there were 22 internationals on the field that day. We had 'em on toast at halftime, then Alf got hurt and the game swung their way. It was do or die the following week against the Bulldogs in the knockout semi. Sometimes an early incident sets the tone of a game. In the 1993 grand final, Saints were psychologically shattered when their top prop Jason Stevens went off in the first minute. A similar decisive moment occurred in the fifth minute of our game against the Bulldogs. Michael Hancock scored an early try from a bomb and we were feeling good. Then, from the restart, Lazzo ran the ball back. He charged into the guts of the Bulldogs forwards. Then *crash!* Dean Pay hit Glenn with a frightening shoulder charge that put Lazzo out of the game with rib cartilage damage. We never recovered and were beaten 24–10.

There was yet more trauma at season's end. The times – and the personnel – were a' changing at the Broncos. Terry Matterson, solid and dependable, an underrated player, departed for the London Broncos. I enjoyed playing with Terry. Julian O'Neill was off too. In spite of scoring eight tries from fullback and 79 goals to be our leading point scorer, he ran out of chances. Julian was sacked from the club after one too many off-field incidents. On the credit side, young

Darren Lockyer was a revelation in his first season with us. In their limited appearances with us, as Wayne eased them into the first grade team, Darren and other young relative unknowns Shane Webcke, Ben Walker, Peter Ryan and Brad Thorn looked like Maroons and Kangaroos of the future. The year was a vast improvement on the two that preceded it, and we were all sure we could go two better in 1996 and bring that Winfield Cup home to Brisbane. Our confidence was misplaced.

Season 1996 started off in the best possible way when Kim fell pregnant with our third child in March. We were living in our beautiful home in Brookfield by then and we couldn't wait for the new addition to the clan. Away from footy, life was bliss. Kim and I had been together for a decade and our love was strong and deep. We were a loving, happy, noisy family about to get even more loving, happier and noisier with the new arrival in December. Looking forward to the blessed event helped me cope with the on-field frustrations and disappointments of 1996, which in many ways mirrored those of the year before. We had a seven-game winning streak early in the season, then rep commitments depleted our side and we lost four out of five in the middle of the year. Mid-season slumps were becoming a regular occurrence. We then recovered to win our last eight competition games straight. We came in second behind Manly in the minor premiership, and went into thc finals with our confidence sky-high, only to lose first to Norths 16–21, then, in the sudden death semi, to Cronulla 16–22.

After being dumped out of the premiership by the Sharks, we felt numb. What had gone wrong? Back then, it didn't seem to us that we were unduly preoccupied by the Super League hassles, but in hindsight it would have been strange if they had not taken some kind of toll. Rugby league is as much a mental as a physical game, and the criticism we copped and the hatred that was directed at our club must have unsettled us. Maybe that turmoil led to the inconsistent form and lack of ball control that hijacked our season. Management laid the blame for our failure at the players' door. Our chairman Paul Morgan agreed that Super League ructions could have derailed us in 1995, but said it was our lack of effort and application that cost us the premiership in 1996. 'We weren't good enough,' he said. 'There were a few holes in the team created by guys who had been there a bit long. Some of them are past their use-by date. I was embarrassed for the players, embarrassed for the people of Brisbane who have supported the team so magnificently for so many years, and embarrassed for the shareholders.' Paul Hauff obviously agreed. He retired that year after playing only a limited number of first grade games, and he said at his farewell presentation that he no longer felt the hunger to train, play and win and suspected that many team-mates didn't either.

I wish I could tell you that things were better in State of Origin, but that was bloody ordinary too. In 1996 the Super League players were eligible for selection again after being banned the year before. But the selectors stuck with most of the young ARL guys and their coach

Paul Vautin who'd won heroically and against the odds in Origin '95. The Broncos traditionally provided 10 or 11 of the Queensland squad, but in this year's series only Alf, Steve Renouf, Wendell Sailor and Brad Thorn were selected in run-on sides, and Alan Cann, Mick Hancock and I – in the second game – warmed the bench. We Super Leaguers felt very much the outsiders, especially when we heard that Fatty had said he'd have been happier to go into the series with an all-ARL team. Fatty denied making the comment.

New South Wales won the opening encounter at Suncorp Stadium 14–6, with Andrew Johns starring. The Blues scrumbase duo of Geoff Toovey and Brad Fittler outplayed Alf and new five-eighth Jason Smith. For Origin II, Alf and Julian O'Neill were at half and five-eighth. I was a reserve. Fatty Vautin brought me into the game late in the first half when we were leading narrowly. He said to me: 'Go out there and change the game.' And I did . . . for NSW. Just before halftime I chip-kicked but the ball corkscrewed into the arms of Laurie Daley who raced 50 metres upfield and passed to Ettingshausen. ET kicked ahead but was impeded by Julian, now at fullback. Penalty to NSW. They declined a shot at goal and kept the pressure on. Furner to ET to Wishart who scored. NSW led at the break and it was all my doing. I didn't even make the bench in Origin III, which NSW won as well to clean-sweep the series.

In rugby league there is a very fine line between being a mug and being a hero. Sometimes it doesn't take a lot to put you off your game. I was very much a confidence player in those days and certainly was upset at being overlooked for Origin I. When I finally got my chance from the bench in the second game, I tried too hard to make things happen. My poorly executed chip was a rash act that backfired. The press had been pushing for my inclusion, saying Alf played so much better when he was partnered with me. But in Origin II at the Sydney Football Stadium even our double act came unstuck. A grim and disappointed Fatty Vautin said afterwards: 'They were all saying Alf Langer goes no good unless Kevin Walters is beside him. The selectors picked him and I put him on after 20 minutes and nothing happened.'

At season's end, Wayne told Kerrod, Willie Carne, Alan Cann and Michael Hancock that they were no longer guaranteed a first grade position with the Broncos and invited them to look for another club. Kerrod was devastated, for he and Wayne went back a long, long way. At first my brother was angry. 'In the early days, the Broncos were 70 per cent a club and 30 per cent a business,' he said. 'Now I think it's the other way around. It's become too business-oriented and I think that's detrimental.' In time, Kerrod came to realise what had happened to him happens to every player. Cutting an ageing player, Wayne told journalist Paul Malone, 'was the process of giving someone else an opportunity, an opportunity the sacked bloke himself received when he was younger. It's a process where, if this club is to remain competitive, it has to be ongoing. There are some who will be able to finish their careers here and there will be some who won't. I don't see it ever changing.' Concerning Kerrod's comment that the Broncos were becoming too hard-headed, he told Malone: 'The players have an obligation to get the job done in football. It's about performance . . . Kerrod would love to be getting $300,000 a year and still have sport as a sport. If he wants it to be a sport, [he should] go back to Ipswich and get $5 a game.'

In the end, Kerrod and Alan Cann joined the new Adelaide Rams team and Willie Carne turned to rugby union. Michael Hancock, always the hardhead who delights in proving others wrong, said he'd take his chances at the Broncos. In 1999 he is still a first grade fixture with us, and when Alf retired in April Michael found himself the last of the original 1988 Broncos team. It was at the end of 1996 when I seriously considered quitting the Broncos and joining brother Steve at North Queensland. Obviously I was upset at how Kerrod had been treated. Wayne talked me out of leaving, and what happened next to Kim and me made me thank God he did.

Normally, at the end of a hard year's footy, Kim, Billy, Jack and I would wind down and relax, enjoy Christmas with the family, take a holiday up the coast, party with the Langers, the Gees, the Lazaruses and the Hancocks. But there was none of that for us that summer, for in August doctors had discovered a lump in my wife's breast. The next 18 months would be spent in a gruelling battle to save Kim's life. Our charmed times were over.

CHAPTER NINE

# LOVE AND LOSS

Kim went to our GP that August morning for her regular smear test. While she was in the surgery, she thought she might as well take the opportunity to tell the doctor about a little soreness she had been feeling in her right breast for about three weeks. She thought it might be a hormonal thing due to the pregnancy. It had only been six months since her last routine breast checkup gave her a clean bill of health. Kim had her breasts examined every 12 months, like clockwork. But this time, after Kim mentioned the soreness, the doctor examined her breast and there was a lump. She sent Kim straight to a specialist at the Wesley Breast Clinic in Brisbane. The appointment was for the very next day. It was quick, they didn't muck around. Kim and I went together and I sat in the waiting room while she was being examined. I thought she'd only be in there for half an hour. Neither of us was worried – you never think anything bad will happen to you, only to others. But when Kim had been in the specialist's room for what seemed to me like bloody hours I began to panic. When she eventually came out she had tears in her eyes. I thought: 'What's going on here?' We went back into the room together, and they took a tissue sample and said they'd have to send it away for tests.

Next morning at training I told my friend Chris Johns what was happening with Kim and he told me not to be too upset. 'Oh, don't worry about it, mate,' he said. 'This stuff happens all the time. I've heard of plenty of women who have had a lump in their breast but it hasn't been cancer.' I was reassured and thought again: 'Cancer won't happen to us.' I arrived home feeling easier, and then Kim told me the tests had revealed that she indeed had a tumour and that they would have to cut her open to see if it was cancerous.

The following afternoon we went to Wesley Breast Clinic for the exploratory surgery. I hugged Kim as she was taken into the operating theatre about 10 o'clock that night and told her everything would be fine. I believed it, too. The doctor assured me he would come and tell me whether or not Kim's tumour was cancerous as soon as he had examined the lump. If it was all clear he would sew Kim up and she'd be out in an hour. If not, if the lump was cancerous, he would perform an immediate lumpectomy – an operation to remove the lump. I was trying to be calm but inside I was panicking. I said: 'Right, fair enough.' The doctor returned to the waiting room an hour later. He said: 'Look, we've got bad news. The lump is cancerous. We have to remove it.' Even then I thought: 'Kevvie, relax. It'll be OK.'

The doctors recommended that Kim undergo chemotherapy at once, to deal with any remaining cancer cells. But she refused point blank. She was terrified that the treatment would harm the baby she was carrying. Who knows, she might have gone on to beat her cancer with immediate chemotherapy, but for Kim that was never an option. I was torn. I didn't know what to do. Kim was flesh and blood, my wife and lover and best friend. Our baby was still only a hope and dream. But Kim had made up her mind. She would have the chemotherapy to save her own life, but not before she gave birth to our third child. She said she had no choice, she was only doing what any mother would do, putting her baby before herself.

Then followed many gruelling sessions with oncologists and paediatricians and it was finally agreed that our baby, who we would call Jett (Kim had read that John Travolta and his wife Kelly Preston had called their son Jett and she liked the name) would be delivered prematurely, at 29 weeks, on 7 October 1996. This was the earliest date, the medicos told us, that our baby could be brought safely into the world, and it was the latest date that Kim could afford to postpone her chemotherapy to and still have a chance of beating her cancer. She would have her breast removed, and then nine months or so later undergo a breast reconstruction operation – in which the doctors take fat tissue from around the stomach and mould it into the shape of a breast and graft it to the chest. Our spirits lifted when we made our plan. We remained confident. The doctors were the best, Kim was healthy and strong and, after all, we still believed, our life was charmed. Remembering those days now, it seems I was in a daze; nothing was real. I had no idea what Kim would have to endure. I never believed for a moment that she could die. Never.

Kim was more realistic than me. She never asked herself: 'Why is this terrible thing happening to me?' She was more of the opinion that: 'These things are part of life. They can strike anyone at any time. Why *not* me?' She got on with what she had to do, accepted that she was ill, that she was pregnant. She would have her baby and then she would have the chemotherapy. We told our families of the situation and they were devastated. We all supported Kim however we could. Her sister Kelly moved in with us to help us look after Jack and Billy. At the Broncos, I told Wayne about Kim, but not too many others. Only my closest friends. I wanted to keep things to myself until Kim and I knew exactly what was going on.

Even though she was often ill and weak, Kim's pregnancy proceeded smoothly, and on 7 October our little blond Jett – who has grown to look very much like his mother – was delivered by caesarean section at Brisbane's Mater Hospital. Kim was conscious for the birth. Then they wheeled her away and anaesthetised her and removed her breast.

She woke up feeling terribly sore, but her only thought was to hold Jett. I remember that, in spite of what had just been done to her, Kimmie was so happy, and I was pushing her around the ward with drips and things hanging out of her body. All she wanted to do was see our baby.

The doctors gave Kim 10 days to regain her strength and let her scars heal and to ensure that there were no infections, and then they started the chemotherapy. Throughout the treatment she'd drag herself to the Mater Hospital twice a day to see Jett in his humidicrib. He remained in hospital until 23 December.

Kim's hair began to fall out. She would wake up in the morning and clumps of hair would be on the pillow. I decided to shave my own head in sympathy. I'm not a pretty guy, so what the hell. The fans – who knew nothing about the tragedy then – must have wondered why I was going for the baldy look. There were other shows of solidarity too. On the night we won the Super League grand final against Cronulla in 1997 at ANZ Stadium, Kim arrived at the post-match celebrations at the Paddington Tavern with sticking plaster on her forehead covering a surgical incision. Janey Dopson came up with the idea of getting the other wives to stick Bandaids on their foreheads too, to show their love and support. Janey reckoned that if anyone asked, they would just say they'd been headbutting each other. There wasn't too much to laugh about in those days, but we all had fun that night. Sure enough, some stranger came up to Kim at the Paddington Tavern and asked: 'What's that lump on your forehead?' And Kim said: 'I'm a champion headbutter! If you want to take me on, you're more than welcome!' And the stranger exclaimed, 'Oh gees, I'm out of here!'

There was another time, earlier in 1997, when a bald Kim came to the party to launch the Broncos' new season and later we went out for a few drinks and a dance, with Glenn Lazarus and Chris Johns and their wives. Well, next day Alf Langer was at the races and a bloke came up to him and said: 'I saw Kevin Walters out drinking last night with a real punky looking chick. She had a shaved head and was dancing all the time. And him, a married man!'

Chemotherapy is bloody awful. It knocked Kim around so badly. She hated losing her hair, but she knew nothing mattered now but staying alive. From the word go, the doctors made it clear that Kim didn't have to have chemotherapy if she didn't want to. She knew it would be a terrible experience. But she understood it was her best chance of survival. We didn't really consider alternative treatment. We were just a normal family and we put ourselves in the hands of the experts. Dr Geoffrey Beadle was excellent, and from the beginning of our nightmare he instilled confidence in us with his expertise and warm authority. He backed Kim in her plan to give birth to Jett, get through the chemotherapy, have a month's rest and then, in July 1997, undergo a breast reconstruction. 'Make plans,' he told her. 'Get on with your life, live as normally as possible and things will fall into place – hopefully.'

Kim had been a smoker all her life, and she took Dr Beadle's advice to live as normally as possible a little too literally. She was feeling much better after the chemotherapy had run its course, and we both dared to hope that she had beaten the cancer. In her optimism she refused to give up cigarettes even though she knew it was essential to do so before she had the breast reconstruction operation. We arrived at the Mater and they put her on a trolley and were about to wheel her into the operating theatre when the doctor smelled tobacco on her breath. 'Have you been smoking?' he demanded. She said: 'Yeah.' 'Then we can't operate,' he said. He cancelled the operation on the spot and told Kim he would proceed when she had been off the smokes for a full week. She stopped smoking right then, but the week's delay meant that I wouldn't be at her side when she went under the knife. I was committed to be in England playing in the Super League World Club Challenge a week from then. I wanted to pull out of the trip but Kim said: 'I'll be fine.' She could have waited a few weeks more for me to arrive home and then had the operation, but she decided she wanted it over and done with as soon as possible. She had her family and mine and Janey there with her so I went overseas with the Broncos. It was all downhill after that.

The four-hour breast reconstruction was winding up in Brisbane as the Broncos plane was landing in England. As soon as I was on the ground I called the hospital and they said the operation had gone fine, that Kim just had a bit of a headache. We'd ring each other twice a day and each time she'd tell me the headache still had not gone away. When I got back home, Kim was just out of hospital and I was alarmed at how she had deteriorated. She was vomiting all the time. I could see her getting worse before my eyes. 'It's back,' I told myself, 'the cancer's back.'

The doctors, however, insisted that it was not. They told us that Kim's lying on her back for four hours throughout the operation could have given her lasting bad headaches. I wasn't convinced and I pumped the doctors with questions and then they did some more tests and took fluid from her spine and sent it away to be analysed. Tragically, I was right. I was sitting in the hospital with some of our family, including Kim's dad Buddy, awaiting the results of the fluid tests, fearing the worst, knowing in my heart that the cancer had escalated in Kim's body. Dr Beadle sat beside me and told me the cancer was now in Kim's spine. Suddenly there was no hope. I accepted for the first time that we were going to lose Kimmie. I was numb with shock. Dr Beadle was saying how breast cancer was treatable and curable but a secondary cancer like she had now was treatable but couldn't be cured. He was saying that Kim was going to die. Later, out of earshot of Buddy and the others, I yelled at Dr Beadle: 'You said, "die"! What is Kim's life expectancy?' He said that in his experience people whose cancer had come back in the spine could expect to live from six to twelve months. 'That's how long Kim has to live?' I screamed.

At first, only Dr Beadle and I knew the terrible prognosis. He thought it best not to tell her, knowing that sufferers of terminal cancer have no illusions. He told me: 'My past experience with patients is that whether you tell them or not they know inside what is happening to their body. If Kim chooses to, she will ask me straight out and I'll be honest with her.' All he said to her that day was: 'The cancer will eventually wear you down.' The doctor instructed me not to tell anyone that Kim would not recover and for a while I didn't. Not my brothers, not my parents, not Kim's parents. Eventually I was going mad being the only one to know. I needed to share our tragedy. So I asked Dr Beadle and he said it would be OK if I confided in Wayne Bennett and Chris Johns. They did everything for me that it was in their power to do. The media did their bit too. Inevitably the newspaper and TV reporters found out about Kim, but they respected our request not to publicise her illness. Guys like Tony Durkin of *Rugby League Week* and Chris Bombolas were truly polite and respectful towards her and her wishes.

Meanwhile, I was as strong as I could be and with Kimmie I kept up my charade that all was well. In September that year, before the Melbourne Cup, she had been feeling a little better, getting around the house OK. So, in an effort to make the most of what time was left to us, I said cheerfully: 'Hey, I have an idea. Let's go to the Melbourne Cup.' She said: 'Why? There's no need to do that. We'll have plenty of opportunities to go to the Cup.' I felt like saying: 'Kim, we won't. Your life will be over in six months!' But of course I didn't, and just mumbled: 'Oh, OK, fair enough.' She only wanted to stay in her beloved home with her beloved boys. I believe that Kim knew she was dying.

Whether she did or not then, she had her sentence confirmed soon afterwards. One night, towards the end of the 1997 season, while I was at the club after a game, she took advantage of my absence to call Dr Beadle and asked him to tell her the truth. 'What's going on with me?' she said. He said simply: 'You'd better come and have a talk with me.' He needed to say no more. She rang the club in tears and told me what Dr Beadle had said, but still I played dumb, pretending that she was on the way to recovery. I hung up and drove straight home. Next day we went to see Dr Beadle and, true to his word, he was honest with Kim. But Kim being Kim, and in spite of the weight of medical opinion against her survival – Dr Beadle said that of all the patients he had treated for cancer of the spine none remained alive – she was adamant that she would beat her cancer. She kept positive even as the treatment intensified, and her attitude was infectious because before long I was convinced that she would survive too and that we'd live happily ever after.

Through all this, Janey Dopson was again proving herself a friend in need. She remarked recently: 'We spent a lot of time together when Kim was sick. It was during the '97 football season and I was pregnant with Michael's and my son, Weston. Kim and I saw each other or spoke on the phone every day, just as we had since we became friends seven years before. Kevin was usually able to take Kim to chemotherapy, but when he was away with the team I'd pack her up and take her to the hospital and stay there with her. In the last few months of her life, we'd sit and talk about anything and everything. We often talked about how the Broncos club was changing as the players who were once young got older, switched clubs or retired. We missed a lot of the wives and girlfriends who had moved on. We also missed our big nights out when we did what we wanted, when we wanted, but by then we all had kids and commitments and Kim had got sick, and those things quieten you down a bit.'

On 6 September the Broncos played the Cronulla Sharks at Stockland Stadium in Townsville in the major semi-final. Kim was in hospital and I rang the doctor and said: 'Look, how is she going?' He replied: 'Not well, but she'll be OK.' And I said: 'There's this big game at the weekend. I really don't want to leave Kim to go up and play. Should I pull out and stay at the hospital? Nothing bad is going to happen, is it?' He replied: 'No, nothing bad is going to happen, I don't think, but I can't guarantee anything. It's best for you to get on with your life.' He was repeating his earlier advice to us to live as normally as possible. I asked Kim what she thought I should do and she said: 'I want you to play. I'm going to be OK. Go up there and have a game of footy.' So I did, and I went to Townsville with Dad and played really well. We won 34–2 and I scored a try.

I was amazed when Kim made it to the 1997 Super League grand final. She'd lost a lot of weight with the chemotherapy because you don't feel like eating and she was sick and fragile from the lumbar punctures and other treatment for her cancerous spine. I was around all the time and what she went through was devastating. It broke my heart. Cancer is so cruel. She'd been in hospital all the week before, but heroically, maybe because she knew it would be the last game she would ever see me play, she dragged herself out of bed to be there. She watched the whole match from the grandstand. I was really proud that she climbed the stairs to have a look. She could only stay at the club for a little while, bravely laughing through her agony, before going home to collapse into bed.

Throughout that year of hell, people were extremely kind to me. Even though I hadn't told all my team-mates of Kim's illness, I learned later that Wayne had got them together and said: 'This is the situation with Kevvie.' He'd told them how ill Kim was, and added: 'And I don't want you moping around here, because that's not what he needs. If he wants to talk to you about it, he'll talk to you. If he doesn't, just try to make him happy and do your best to be as normal as possible.' Everybody at the Broncos rallied around. I'd turn up at training with my jaw on the ground and they'd pick me up through their friendship and their love for Kim and me which shone through these macho guys in spite of themselves.

All year, footy was a welcome distraction from the tragedy unfolding at home. Without it I would have gone mad. Season 1997 was the year when Australian rugby league split in two: an ARL competition comprising the eventual premiers, Newcastle, and Manly, Balmain, Gold Coast, Illawarra, Norths, Parramatta, St George, South Queensland, Souths, Sydney City and Wests; and a Super League comp, the Telstra Cup, fought out by the Broncos, Adelaide, Auckland, Canberra, Canterbury, Cronulla, Hunter, Penrith and Perth. In direct contrast to the unsettled and divisive 1995 and 1996 seasons, we did it all that year. We lost only three games out of the 29 Telstra Cup premiership and World Cup Challenge games we played. We won every home match. In the grand final we were too strong for Cronulla, winning 26–8.

A highlight for me was our first-half performance against Cronulla in the major semi when we racked up 30 points against them with the precision Broncos football of old. We had cricket scores against the best British Super League clubs: 34–0 against Wigan, 76–0 against Halifax, 66–12 against St Helens when Steve Renouf scored five tries. The decline of these once-great and proud English teams was saddening. Against the Sharks, we were hot. It was the Broncos at their best.

On the other side of the footy ledger, Queensland was pipped 23–22 by New South Wales in the final of the inaugural Super League Tri-State series. And we lost Lazzo. Glenn broke his leg playing in the British section of the World Club Challenge campaign and never played for the Broncos again. Wayne decided that we could no longer afford him under the salary cap. He was nearing 30 then, but still the best prop in the world. He is still playing for Australia and captaining the Melbourne Storm as I write this in 1999.

Also, Kerrod was no longer with us. I was rocked when he was cut from the team at the end of 1996 and joined Adelaide. For a while – until Wayne talked me out of it and I realised that taking Kim far from the medical facilities of Brisbane was not a good idea – I considered leaving the Broncos in protest and joining my brother Steve, who was bound for North Queensland after years with the Raiders. I loved playing with Kerrod and he was still, in my opinion, playing top footy. He agonised over being shown the door. He couldn't understand how they could kick him out of the club after he'd been our best forward in the finals series. Wayne simply told him: 'Pack your bags and away you go.' I think the club management, and especially John Ribot who I believe had never been a fan of Kerrod, was looking to make changes. Ben Walker, John Plath and John Driscoll are excellent players, but I still didn't think there was a hooker in the club as good as my brother, but maybe I was biased. I guess, too, my itchy feet were also a result of realising that my own place in the team was being threatened by a number of brilliant youngsters who had come to the Broncos. In the end, I decided to stay and repel the challengers.

I hadn't been impressed in 1996 when our new recruit for 1997, Anthony Mundine, paraded in a Broncos jumper for the TV cameras while he was still contracted to St George – and not just because I thought it was poor form and a very unprofessional and un-Broncos-like sideshow. Mundine made it clear that he had set his sights on my five-eighth spot in the Brisbane backline, the position I had held since I took over from Wally Lewis in 1990. Choc is one of the most natural athletes ever to play our game. He is a superbly balanced runner and passer of the ball, a beautiful footballer who'll play for Australia. He is also one of the most controversial guys in league and rarely out of the headlines. He is supremely confident in his ability, gamely criticising greats like Laurie Daley who, he said, was 'running on old legs'. He is not afraid to make waves if he feels he is right, such as when he refused to turn the other cheek when he believed he had been racially vilified by Canterbury's Barry Ward. Unfortunately for Choc, he was unable to dislodge me at the Broncos. He played a lot of centre for us in 1997, and returned to the Saints in 1998, grizzling that he had not been treated like royalty in Brisbane.

Somehow, in spite of my constant heartbreak over Kim, I had a vintage year in football in 1997. Perhaps Wayne believed that added responsibility at the Broncos would distract me, if only a little, from personal agonies. I took over as skipper when Alf was injured and had a perfect captaincy record. I was runner-up to my old sparring partner Peter Ryan as the Broncos player of the year. The tragedy was affecting me in ways I can't even now explain. One Friday afternoon, after getting some bad news about Kim, I went to training and I ran the fastest time – by far – I've ever run. It was an 8 km course and I ran so fast, it was like I was getting strength and speed from a source outside myself. Like running with a gale behind my back. Perhaps all the emotions I was experiencing did something to my adrenalin. I think I still hold the club record for that run.

I made myself unavailable to play for Australia if

selected in the three-Test Super League series against Great Britain in England because I didn't want to leave Kim and the boys. Wayne seemed satisfied with what I'd delivered in 1997. 'Kevvie was sensational for us this year,' he told *Rugby League Week* at the season's end. 'Even though Alf is the designated skipper, Kevvie does a lot of the leading out there. He often calls the shots, and does it superbly. But this past season he was literally left on his own when both Alf and Lazzo were injured in England in July. Lazzo didn't play again and Alf did as much as he could under extreme discomfort, but the hard, cold facts were that Kevvie became our hardhead out there in the middle for the later part of the season. I will never underestimate the job he did for us.'

Jack, Billy and Jett, too, kept me going in 1997. Their love and reliance on me held me together when inside I felt I was coming apart and I was doing it tough to put one foot in front of the other. One thing is true about little boys: they keep you busy. Then, and today with Kim gone, there are times when it would be easy to hit the bottle or lock myself away in a room and cry all day, but my boys mean I will never do that. If not for them, I may have gone around the bend.

As Kim's disease progressed she was wasting away in front of our eyes, and one night it became clear to us that our days of pretending that there would be a happy ending to her struggle were over. We took the kids out to a Sizzler restaurant at Kenmore, near our home, and Kim was talking about Jett's hair – how it had started to go curly. 'Don't you cut his hair off until it's really long,' she told me. I said: 'What do you mean?' I didn't cut the boys' hair, Kim did. She said: 'Well, I might not be around in two or three years time.' And we both started crying in the middle of this bloody Sizzler. We both just sat there on our stools and bawled. But not for very long. Then we had a cuddle and a hug and soon we were laughing. Saying at last what both of us had been afraid to come out and say made it easier for us to map out a future for our boys without their mum.

We never told the boys that Kim had cancer, just that she had some germs in her body and the doctors were trying to get them out and that's why she was in and out of hospital all the time. I didn't take them to the hospital too much. When Kim was up to it, we discussed how we wanted Jack, Billy and Jett to live their lives, their schooling, what kind of men we wanted them to grow up to be. One thing we knew: we didn't want the boys growing up feeling sorry for themselves because they didn't have a mother. You see so many children who lose a parent to illness or an accident or through divorce, and those kids turn into brats. We didn't want that to happen to our sons and my goal in life is to bring up the boys as good and loving men.

We'd put aside photo albums and videos of Kim for our family to cherish and remember her by. At Christmas, 1997, just a few weeks before she died, Kim wrote letters to Jack, Billy and Jett. In each letter she said goodbye and told them what they meant to her. They're not allowed to open their letter until they're old enough to read it and understand. She told me that writing those letters was the hardest thing she ever did in her life. Harder than the chemotherapy and anything else her cancer put her through. Nothing was as daunting as sitting down and putting pen to paper for the boys, knowing that she wasn't going to be around forever and a day.

In early November, Peter Jackson was found dead. Kim thought the world of Peter, having known him since our Canberra years. She made a monumental effort to drag herself to his memorial service on the beach at Stanwell Park, south of Sydney. As I've said, it was a serene ceremony, a celebration of this wonderful joker's life, but it was heavy with portents of more grieving to come. I walked away from Jacko's funeral, sad that we'd lost him but feeling good that the service was so well done. It went off beautifully. Knowing in my heart what would almost certainly happen to Kim in the next months, I decided that I would give her a funeral as tasteful and touching as Jacko's.

For Kim, the end came with a rush. I could see she was getting sicker. Earlier she might have gone three or four weeks between visits to the hospital, then it was two weeks, and then she had to go every week. After the cancer reappeared in her spine I saw her gradually slide away from us. She had no doubts about what awaited her. She composed the letters, and then she wrote in a book instructions about who she wanted to leave her rings and jewellery and other precious things to. She asked that the gifts she had received since she fell ill be returned to the people who gave them to her. Looking back, I guess we were blessed that we had a chance to make our plans. So many people lose their life suddenly, just like that, in a car accident or whatever. We were lucky because we had time to say goodbye.

In the final weeks of her illness, Kim would lie all day in bed or on the lounge, racked by pain in her body and the headaches. She was too sick even to watch TV. She was on a lot of morphine and bombed-out much of the time. Even then, her sense of humour did not fail her. She got a big Tupperware bowl and wrote on it 'Kim's Spew Bucket'. That spew bucket was her constant companion. She carried it wherever she went. She vomited constantly. It was an awful way to live. She was furious that she was too sick to look after the boys. She wanted to mother them but she could not. That hurt her as much as anything. When her condition grew so bad that she had to be hospitalised, her sister Kelly and I would take turns sleeping in a little room outside her bedroom; the other one would be at home with Jack, Billy and Jett.

The Wesley doctors and nurses were wonderful to us. If there can be such a thing as a 'good' hospital, given all the suffering that goes on in those places, then the Wesley is certainly one. Going to that hospital helped me to stop feeling sorry for myself. A couple of times I found myself thinking: 'Why have we been singled out for this suffering?' Then I'd get into a lift at the Wesley and there would be a little girl, eight years old, no hair, going through chemotherapy for leukaemia, and I'd realise that there is always someone worse off than yourself.

Kim was in hospital for the three or four days leading up to Christmas Day 1997 and was determined to get home for the 25th. It was very important to her to be at home with the boys that day. It was a job convincing the doctors that she could check herself out, but we managed, and she had to inject herself in the stomach with morphine to stand the pain. We arrived home on the evening of Christmas Eve. She had a *horrible* night. She could hardly sleep at all, up all the time taking drugs, me preparing the mixtures for her. But when the boys woke up on Christmas morning, there she was to greet them with a big smile. And you should have seen the smile on *their* faces. Enormous! I'll never forget her bravery.

In January 1998 Kim and I were out briefly, shopping for school uniforms and schoolbooks in Brisbane, when she got dizzy and faint. We went straight home. That night, around one o'clock, Kim tried to get out of bed to go to the toilet and collapsed onto the floor. I helped her to the toilet and she was vomiting everywhere. I raced her straight to hospital. She never came home.

For ten days Kim lapsed in and out of consciousness. For a few hours now and then we talked and cried and occasionally laughed. She reiterated how she wanted me to raise Jack, Billy and Jett, how she wanted them to be loved and cared for. She stressed the importance of a good education. She said she wanted always to be remembered. 'I love you,' she told me. 'And be strong for the boys.'

I refused to take Billy, Jack and Jett to visit Kim in

hospital at the end. I didn't want them to see her in that condition. It was a terrible decision to have to make. It meant depriving them of saying a last goodbye to their mum, but in the end I kept them home. I wanted them to remember Kim as she was before she got sick, as a beautiful person who loved them dearly and did everything for them, rather than this pale woman lying in a bed scarcely able to lift an eyelid.

For me there was something so strong about her spirit that, in spite of all her suffering, in spite of the way the cancer destroyed her, when I think of Kim now – as I do every day – I don't remember her ill and ravaged, I remember her beautiful and well and happy.

At last, as the pain grew worse and more and more morphine was administered, Kim sank into unconsciousness. With my grief, I also felt relief. From the day she was diagnosed with cancer in August 1996, I reckon she had only had about one month when she wasn't ill or in pain or in hospital or had no hair or no breast or wasn't taking drugs. At last, now, her ordeal was drawing to a close. Dr Beadle said, as Kim slipped further and further away from us: 'This is probably going to be the end.' I rang my family in Ipswich and Kim's in Toowoomba and told them to hurry to the hospital. We were all gathered around her bed when Kim died at 5.30 a.m. on Friday, 6 February 1998.

The day was dawning grey and overcast as I drove home to be with the boys. I sat them down in the loungeroom and, armed with advice I'd read in a Queensland Cancer Fund book which explains how birds, trees and butterflies and all living things must die, I told them Kim was gone. A terrible task: how do you tell your children that they will never see their mother again? It was bloody awful. We cried and cried, not so much Jett because he was still a baby, but Jack and Billy. Then, after five minutes, Billy said: 'Dad, can we go out and kick the footy now?' So he, also, was too young then to appreciate what had happened. Not so Jack. He knew, and was then, and still is, affected by Kim's death.

It sounds like a strange thing to do, perhaps, but after we'd visited Kim's parents at home in Toowoomba we returned to Kelvin Grove that afternoon and I trained with the Broncos, and took the boys along too. I was still in shock and consumed by sadness and I simply needed people around me. I didn't want to be alone.

In the days that followed, we were deluged with flowers and cards and letters from friends and strangers. The joint was like a florist shop for two or three months. The house was filled, and so were our hearts. I have a box on my mantelpiece and in it I keep every card and letter that was sent to me. Kim's sister Kelly, Janey Dopson and I had thank-you cards printed and we sent one to everybody who'd expressed their feelings.

The funeral was held on the morning of 9 February at St Luke's Church of England in Toowoomba. Four hundred mourners packed the church: our families, friends, a big footy contingent including Wayne Bennett, Glenn Lazarus, Darren Lockyer, Michael Hancock and all my Broncos team-mates, and Chris

Johns, Wally Lewis, John Ribot, Gene Miles, Trevor Gillmeister, Laurie Daley, John Plath and Wendell Sailor. Peter Jackson's still-grieving widow Siobhan was there. Only months earlier I had been mourning her lost spouse, now she was mourning mine. Just as Kim, ever the organised one, had prepared for the welfare of our boys, so she had made plans for the funeral. She had made me promise to have played during the service the songs that meant so much to her. Daryl Braithwaite's 'Horses' was for Jack and Billy, and Savage Garden's 'Truly, Madly, Deeply' was for Jett, for this was the song she sang to him in the car. Boz Scaggs' 'Fly like a Bird' was broadcast for her dad. 'Say a Little Prayer', for Kim's sister Rach, and 'Beautiful Sunday' rang out through the old church. Celine Dion's ballad 'Because You Love Me' was her special gift to me that day.

Wayne Bennett spoke to the congregation. 'We all learn how to live,' he said, 'but Kim taught us how to die – with great dignity, with humour, conquering her fear.'

And somehow, through my tears, I delivered a eulogy I had written in the days before. My voice quavered as I read it out:

> Although Kim and I went to school together at Bremer State High School in Ipswich we never really met until we were seventeen years old. I was immediately attracted to her natural beauty and elegance. You could say she was a glamour. But she was only human, and before long we were dating

and virtually inseparable. However, I still had one hurdle to overcome – his name was Buddy Facer, Kim's dad. Everyone knew of his boxing talents and his particular dislike of any young man showing interest in his prized possession. So Kim and I had to put a game plan together. Because we were both working, the only time we got to spend together was at night, after I had finished footy training. I would race home, have a quick shower, something to eat and speed off to Kim's place at McGregor Street in Ipswich. Kim and I decided that the best way for me to avoid this giant of a man was to turn off my car lights – and the motor – at the top of the hill, and then roll down the street to her driveway. Her bedroom was downstairs, so it was a quick sprint into her room, and safety. Buddy tells me today that he knew what was going on. He just had a hunch that our relationship would be long-term. And he was right.

In 1986 I received an offer to play with Canberra. I didn't even get a chance to ask Kim if she would accompany me. She had begun packing already. We could not have been happier. Kim had many special qualities. She was always positive toward my football career, and this was extremely important for any young player trying to make it in rugby league. Many a night I would come home from training complaining about something, and she would turn the position or situation around for me and get me positive and enthusiastic again.

We returned to Brisbane in 1990. Our three years

in Canberra had been a great experience and a learning curve for us both, but it was nice to be back with our respective families. We were married a year later in 1991, and were excited about the prospect of starting a family of our own. I am so grateful she has given me three beautiful and lovable boys, and there is no doubt Kim has left a mark on each of our sons. Jack has her determination, Billy has her temper and Jett has her easygoing nature. Of course, they inherited their good looks from their dad.

Kim could see good things in any situation. Before she passed away we were fortunate enough to discuss the children's future, and I promise you, Kim, that all your wishes will be put in place as time goes by.

These past eighteen months have been very difficult for everyone concerned, but none more so than Kim herself. She has continually been brave, unselfish and loving under the most trying conditions. Never once did I hear her complain or whinge about her illness. Sorry, there *was* one time – she wasn't very happy about not being able to have a smoke in her room at the hospital.

As the disease began to take its toll, I found myself getting stronger with her. Kim had an unbelievable inner strength, and I will take this strength that she has given me into the battles which lie ahead in my life. I truly felt privileged to be able to care for and nurture such a wonderful human being. She taught me many a lesson throughout this terrible ordeal.

There are obviously many people to thank for their love and support over the years, especially Buddy and Rhonda and all the Facer family. Kim was worried about you, Buddy, from the time she was diagnosed until her death. About how you would handle things. But you showed your greatness all the way through, and I thank you for that. The boys at the Broncos have made you an honorary member at our annual end-of-season drink. All you have to do is make sure the hair on your chest grows back. To Lorraine, Kim's mum, thanks heaps. We couldn't have survived this without your support. I'm hoping the boys will see plenty more of you. To KG and Sandy, my parents – and all members of the Walters family – you have all been a tower of strength for me and the kids. I feel at ease with the love and strength you all showed me and the boys. Janey Dopson has been a loyal and true friend to Kim for nine years now . . . She is part of a select group of people who I could call on, and trust, without hesitation. Thanks, Janey. Last, but by no means least, there is Kim's sister Kelly, or Rach as she is better known. Way back when Kim first fell ill and we needed help on a permanent basis, Rach dropped everything and came running into our lives with open arms.

These are just a few of the many, many people who have been wonderful to me, Kim and the boys. I hope and pray that this support network will continue on for all of us.

The time has come for us all to say goodbye to

Kim. My past thirteen years with you, Kim, have been a treat. We experienced plenty of highs and a few lows, and all those memories will stay with me forever. After seeing first-hand what you have been through, I'm now at ease knowing that my beautiful, unselfish, loving wife and mother of my boys is now resting in peace.

You will never be forgotten. I love you, Kim. Goodbye. God bless.

Afterwards there was a small wake in Toowoomba, but I didn't linger. I drove back to Brisbane with the boys that evening. I didn't want to have a drink. Alcohol can bring on a lot of emotions and I didn't want to get myself into that situation. All I wanted to do was to be at home with my sons and reflect on the wonderful life Kim and I had shared.

CHAPTER TEN

# KIM'S LEGACY

Kim was one of the six women who die of breast cancer every day in Australia. That's one life lost to the disease every four hours. In our country, one in every 12 women are affected by breast cancer.

While she was undergoing treatment Kim was invited to attend a meeting of women who either had breast cancer or were in remission from it. She told me how she found strength talking with these women. They made her feel that she wasn't alone. She was inspired by them, and also realised how important it was for sufferers to receive emotional support and good advice from people who have been touched by the disease. She said her dream was to set up an ongoing and well-organised program where women could come and speak and listen in a group situation. Where they could support each other. From first-hand experience, Kim knew that cancer can affect you emotionally as well as physically and she realised the need for psychological care as well as medical treatment. She once told me: 'When I beat this bloody cancer, I'm going to counsel women who have the disease. I'm going to help them, like other women helped me. That's why I've been put on earth. I know it.'

Kim died before she could realise her plan, but happily now her dream is coming true. After Kim passed away, *New Idea* magazine called me wanting to do a story. I was a bit iffy. My emotions were still raw and I didn't think I could get through an interview without falling to pieces. But when *New Idea* (as part of their bid to raise $1.25 million to fight breast cancer across Australia) offered to donate $10,000 towards setting up Kim's program, I said to the magazine: 'Let's do it.' I knew the most deserving recipient would be the Wesley Hospital which ran a service, the Choices Program, that offered practical advice, emotional support and counselling for women with breast cancer and for their families. That dovetailed with what Kim wanted to set up. I spoke with Dr Cherrell Hirst, director of the Wesley Breast Clinic, and Wesley's director of community relationships, Ray Crompton, and in March 1998, a month or so after Kim's death, the Wesley's Choices Program became the Kim Walters Choices Program, in memory of Kim. I would be a hands-on patron and vowed to finish the job my wife started.

Today the Kim Walters Choices Program is going like hellfire. It's a free, walk-in counselling service, no appointment necessary, providing information and emotional support for women sufferers and their families. They hold meetings at the Wesley Breast Clinic and on Mondays in the boardroom at the Broncos Leagues Club, but there are plans to make the service available every day, and there will be branches at Logan City and Ipswich by the end of 1999. The atmosphere is friendly, informal and relaxed. At the Program, breast cancer sufferers and their loved ones can speak to each other and hear the wisdom of professional cancer counsellors and doctors. The Program is staffed by Wesley Breast Clinic nurses and counsellors and volunteers from the Friends of The Wesley Breast Clinic, most of whom have had breast cancer and have received extensive and comprehensive training to enable them to talk with other sufferers. It is a community service for women of all walks of life. Kim would be proud knowing that these ladies are getting help and that their families are being supported when they need it most. The Program pays for the services of the experts, and if a sufferer is referred to a psychologist, for instance, it pays for that too. Terry Mudie, chief executive of the Wesley Hospital, says of the Program: 'It helps women make choices in dealing with breast cancer, acknowledges that a woman needs treatment as a whole, not just surgery or radiation therapy – and if depression or anxiety is identified, the appropriate added care can be provided. Kevin and his family have done an enormous service to the Queensland community by giving Kim's name to this free counselling service.'

The club venue gives people a chance to get away

from hospitals. It's good to see so many men at the meetings. Husbands often think it's not macho to talk about their grief and fears, to speak to someone about their loved one's illness. They say: 'I'll be OK. I can get through this on my own.' I know that when I learned to confide in others and not be too scared to reach out to get help, it made coping with Kim's illness easier.

Dr Hirst is right when she says that we all live our life on four planes – physical, intellectual, emotional and spiritual – and that they are all entwined. The medical world all too often forgets this and focuses on the medical treatment and neglects the other planes. Surgery, chemotherapy and other treatment are vital, but often not enough. 'For women with breast cancer, one of the most important steps is to have the opportunity to speak openly, honestly, but also privately, about issues that confront them,' Dr Hirst maintains.

Lorna Cook, a Friend of The Wesley Breast Clinic, had one breast removed 20 years ago and the other 10 years later. She knows only too well that knowledge and support are the essential links between illness and rehabilitation for many sufferers of breast cancer. When she had her mastectomies, she said, no one would speak openly with her about what she was going through. It took her 18 months to get over the trauma of losing a body part and during that time no one gave her support based on first-hand experience. At the Choices Program, Lorna is one of many people giving sufferers the benefit of her experience.

Recent research published in *The Medical Journal of Australia* proves that Lorna, Dr Hirst – and Kim, who came to know how vital emotional support for breast cancer sufferers can be – are on the right track. Professor David Kissane of Melbourne University's Centre for Palliative Care and Dr David Clarke of Monash University's Psychological Medicine Department examined the psychological state of 303 women recently diagnosed with early breast cancer. Nearly half of these women – about 42 per cent – had developed depression or anxiety, or both. The rate is twice that of women in the general population. Of the 42 per cent suffering psychiatric disorders, 37 per cent had depression, 10 per cent had major depression, 9 per cent had an anxiety disorder and 7 per cent a phobic disorder. The women suffered fatigue and reduced physical activity, were resigned that they would die, or blocked out the issue completely. They had negative moods, including a sense of hopelessness. Some 84 per cent of the women had lost interest in sexual activity, 29 per cent felt less attractive, 15 per cent felt less feminine, and 13 per cent were dissatisfied with their body. Professor Kissane said there was a need for improved psychological support for women once they were diagnosed. 'A lot needs to be done to bring the delivery of high quality support services up to par to help women make the adjustments involved.'

The Program is funded by donations from the public and through fundraising events. In 1998 we raised $35,000 from the sale of pink ribbons with the name of our charity and the Wesley's logo (a cross) imprinted on them, and we hope to make more than that this year during Pink Ribbon Fortnight. I get along to every meeting I can. I keep my finger on the pulse and know exactly how it's faring. Right now, the Program is confined to Queensland, with counselling centres about to open in Ipswich and Logan, but there are plans to take it national. Still, I'm very concerned that we do things correctly rather than expanding half-cocked. Let's get our own backyard in order first. Wayne Bennett and other Broncos players have been along to fundraisers and Janine Langer, Andrew Gee's wife Sharon and Janey Dopson have rolled up their sleeves and been very supportive.

At the March 1998 launch of the Kim Walters Choices Program, I joked that helping to set up the Program gave me an even bigger buzz than beating Manly, but I hope no one mistook my one-liner for any lack of serious intent. From the very start, people and organisations throughout Queensland pitched in, and nowhere were ordinary citizens more enthusiastic than in Ipswich. In July, the First Provincial Building Society there donated $1000 and sold pink ribbons over the counter, while one of my old stamping grounds, the Star Tavern, handed over $4370 from a fundraising dinner in June attended by 130. The Star's assistant manager Brett Mackay called Kim's Program 'a good cause, and with Kevvie being a local lad, it was just a great opportunity to help'. After the Star Tavern turnout, one Jan Ackroyd Bailey wrote to the local paper saying she herself had survived breast cancer and thanked the function's organisers for a night of 'good food, good entertainment and good fellowship'. The Ipswich Youth Council screened *A Bug's Life* at Ipswich City Cinema and the proceeds from ticket sales were donated to us.

Elsewhere, prize-winning Redcliffe gardener Val Head opened her garden to the public in September and gave the money paid at the gate by garden-lovers, $3.50 a head, to the Program. 'I had a friend and a cousin who both died from breast cancer and I know how tragic it can be, so I decided I would like my garden to help women at the Wesley,' she said. Men rallied to the cause. Truck drivers, builders, railway workers and businessmen forked out. The Wesley's business program manager Kathryn McKewin was blown away by their generosity and noted how it was unusual for 'the traditional blokey' sector of the community to donate money to a breast cancer fund. But, she added, 'Kim's death was so heart-rending that men are realising it's not just women who suffer, but the whole family.'

Capalaba women Kym Sears and Kathy Beale came up with a handy method of raising funds. They took plaster casts of the hands of Broncos players and auctioned them to fans. 'It's amazing how much money some fans will spend following their players to games all over the country,' said Kym. 'So we thought they would probably be more than happy to be able to buy their favourite player's handcast.' So it turned out, and Kim's Program and the Sudden Infant Death Syndrome Program benefited. Then there was the dance at Tamrookum Hall, Beaudesert, organised by a good-hearted local, Mac Smith. Bands played for free, people brought a plate of food and the $6 admission charge went to the Program. Everyone had a ball and they raised $600. At Stones Corner, the Rotary Art

Show gave us $5500 raised from the sale of paintings. Buderim residents Kerrie and Livio Piva presented a 'wonderland of lights' display for the community at their home, and the spectacular show brought us $1139.50.

When the Broncos played Melbourne Storm in July at ANZ Stadium in one of the big premiership matches of 1998, it was designated 'The Official Kim Walters Choices Program Charity Game' and the charity's name was emblazoned on the playing field. We asked the 35,119 fans who turned up to buy a pink ribbon for $2. They came to the party and the Program's coffers swelled by more than $25,000 that night. There was a special telephone donation line. It made me glow with pride to see how footy followers got behind the Program, and I'll remember as long as I live how they gave me a special cheer when I crossed for one of our tries in the Broncos' 34–16 victory. Kim could not have been remembered in a nicer way.

That season, too, the Broncos Supporters Group raised $300 by raffling a Brisbane jersey. The supporters, the players, their wives and the cheer squad all got involved. Janey Dopson, Janine Langer and Sharon Gee, who had joined the Program's committee, were interviewed by a reporter, Christine Sams. 'Janey and Kim's bond was lovely and touching,' said Janine. Janey agreed: 'In a lifetime, you probably find a couple of examples of true friendship and Kim was a true friend to me. When she became ill, her true colours really shone through and her strength and courage inspired us all.' The three declared that they would carry on Kim's commitment to help fellow sufferers by serving on the committee. 'Kim was always very positive she was going to beat her cancer,' said Sharon. 'I was inspired by her attitude to try to fulfil her dreams of helping other women.' And Janine said: 'Kim's death was sad in so many ways, but we were lucky to have shared time with her. We'll cherish that for the rest of our lives.'

The only rule about fundraising functions at the Wesley is that they must be the type of function Kim would be proud to attend. As Kim's dad, Buddy Facer, says: 'Kathryn McKewin said any function we hold will be clean-cut, no dirty jokes, no Rodney Rude-type fellas, because Kim was an angel.'

In March 1999, one year after the charity kicked off, Queensland health minister Wendy Edmond got right behind the program when she declared our Pink Ribbon Corporate Campaign open at the Wesley Hospital. Executives and administrators from more than 150 business and sporting organisations turned up. I spoke at the function. 'I know that a lot of women are being helped and supported by the Wesley Hospital in the way Kim would have liked,' I assured the throng. 'I especially thank the Wesley Hospital, the Brisbane Broncos, *New Idea* and all those who meet with me each month to help plan the fundraising activities of the program – particularly those volunteers who give of their time so freely.'

The more money we raise, the more sufferers of breast cancer we can help. I think Kim would be happy with her Program's progress so far.

CHAPTER ELEVEN

# HEART SONGS

We miss Kim every day, but we miss her most on special days like her birthday, Christmas Day and Mother's Day, when all the kids at school make little gifts to give their mum. This year we found a solution: Jack and Billy made presents for their grandma. I feel extremely sad for the boys' sake. It must be awful for them on days such as these. It really does make me sad. But we must push through the tough days and look forward to happier times.

We've had some difficult times with Jack since Kim passed away. He has taken her death hard, but at the moment he's going good and handling himself wonderfully well. I think that's due to his mother and the way she brought him up. He's a likeable lad, very smart and switched on for his age. Jack looks like me – poor little bugger – but Billy and Jett are very much their mother's sons and often people say to me: 'Gee! Look at those two, the spitting image of Kim.' I swell with pride. Jack is very much a thinker, as Kim was. He never rushes into things and always thinks about what he's doing. Billy has definitely inherited Kim's temper. His moods change constantly. One minute he's as happy as Larry; next minute I say, 'Stop kicking the ball in the house', and he goes off his brain. He doesn't like being told what to do. Neither did Kim. Jett is laidback, nothing too much seems to faze him. Kim was usually that way too. They're all a mixture of our various ways. Other personality traits may emerge as they grow older. But one thing is for sure: I see my sons and know that Kim is well and truly still with us.

I'm coping as well as can be expected. I've always been a hands-on dad and tried to involve myself with my kids. I could never be the sort of father who doesn't come home and fobs off his kids when they want to play. I do a lot of what I want to do these days, and not so much of what other people expect me to do. Now, without Kim, my job has intensified. I try to be dad and mum, but that's not possible and I need help and support. So many people have put their hands up to lend assistance. At times the boys are very demanding, like all kids, and I think: 'Oh, gee, guys, give me a break. Let me go and do this or that.' But if I'm away for a night playing footy and come home and the boys are not in the house I think: 'Where are they? Bring 'em home!'

Since Kim's death I've tried to raise the boys pretty much as we brought them up together. I play with them a lot, make them feel special. We eat breakfast and dinner together. We've always been close, so I don't think I'm guilty of smothering them. It can be hard to find that happy medium. I haven't really tried to compensate for Kim by taking them to over-the-top outings. We've been to Dreamworld on the Gold Coast a couple of times. I take them to Toowoomba to see their granddad Buddy, and they punch the bag in his gym. They love kicking the footy around – and that's not something that's been rammed down their throats. They enjoy it. Jack plays with his cousins and does just fine but I don't care what sport they play so long as they get their teeth into something, whether it's rugby league or tennis or golf or music. Jack's had a crack at soccer. Fine by me.

The boys come to the Broncos games and will happily sit and watch me play so long as they have a bucket of chips and a can of Coke in their hands. After games at ANZ Stadium they're allowed to run onto the field and have a boot around with the kids of the other Broncos. Mum and Dad help a lot on match days. When I'm getting ready to play, they make sure the kids are OK in the stand. When I played for Australia in 1998, the boys came to camp and I introduced them to their favourites, Andrew Johns, Tim Brasher and Ben Ikin. They know all the players from TV. Jack is now a ballboy for the Broncos. He had his first game in our opening match of the 1999 season against Cronulla. I was coming off the field at halftime and it was hot and we were getting flogged and I had a hundred worries racing through my head. I saw Jack and I went over to him and I put my arm around him and said: 'G'day, Jack. How ya goin'?' He said: 'Not good, Dad.' 'Why, mate?' 'Well,' he said, 'someone stole my bloody sandbucket!' That brought me right back to reality. I was worried sick about how we were going to turn things around against the Sharks, and this little kid . . . his biggest drama was that someone had stolen his sandbucket. I laughed inside and thought: 'Well, gee – what are we on this earth for!' Sometimes I think we adults take things too seriously. We'd all do better to sit back and relax a little more and see the world through the eyes of kids. I got a few smiles after a deeply disappointing match when I was copping some flak for passing the ball over the head of our winger straight into touch. 'But Jack called for it!' I protested.

It's no big deal to Jack that his dad plays for the Broncos. Sometimes I'm not sure that the boys even realise I'm a first grade rugby league player. They sure don't treat me like a star! About the only time Jack has acknowledged that I've got a public profile is when he said: 'Dad, when we go the shops, how come everyone knows your name? Why can't they just leave you alone?' It's not as if I get mobbed in the street like Alf, but one day I said: 'Come on, mate. We'll go to the shops and have a milkshake and something to eat.' He said: 'Yeah, I'll go, but please don't sign any autographs today.'

Three boys are going to be a handful for me for many years to come. The temptations and dangers that await my sons chill me to the bone. But I'm ready for 'em and I'm looking forward to us all growing up together. I'm content with what we have and where we're going. It has not been easy since Kim's death, because she was a superb mother. I'm grateful for all the happy years we had together. We may have lost Kim in a physical sense, but we haven't lost her in any other way. She is still around us all the time, looking over us.

We love our home here at Brookfield. There's plenty of room for growing boys to spread out. It's rural although only 20 minutes from the city. I'm grateful Kim got twelve months or so to live here, but it's so sad that she can't enjoy all the years of work she put in when we were struggling to afford to live in such a lovely home. That's one of the saddest things. Still, look around the house and there are memories of her in every room. There are photographs of Kim and letters and all kinds of treasures and objects she left us. We're surrounded by things that are important to us. All my football mementoes are on the walls: my Kangaroo, Queensland and Broncos jumpers, trophies and photos of the great games. Even more important, every surface is covered with family photos. Kim is everywhere. And there's the tree. In March 1998 we planted a tree in the backyard in Kim's memory. I went to the local nursery and said: 'I need a tree that is going to grow tall and give long-term shade.' We planted it and the kids and I tend it. It's growing strong.

Just before she passed away, Kim told the boys that if they ever needed to reach out to her they must go outside and look up into the sky and find the brightest star. That will be her. Many times they've cried for their mummy, so out we go onto the front verandah and find that star and we have a bit of a chat with Kim. They tell her what's going on and what they've been doing.

Super League has given me a degree of financial security, and I'm grateful for that. It means we have private health insurance, which was a blessing when Kim was sick because her medical bills were astronomical. It means I can afford to have a terrific nanny for the boys in Cara Weily, who answered an ad and has become an important part of our lives. I couldn't do without her. For eight weeks after Kim died, Mum and Dad moved in with us, and that was good and they were badly needed, but I knew that after a couple of weeks it was time for them to go home to Ipswich and for us to make it on our own. I didn't want Mum and Dad, who are meant to be enjoying life's luxuries now, to be tied up with Jack, Billy and Jett at the expense of all my brothers' children. Kids need grandparents to spoil them.

Cara Weily was the first person to respond to my ad for a nanny to look after Jack, Billy and Jett. Janey Dopson and I interviewed her and something clicked right away. She was right, and the job was hers. She told me she had been driving and had heard about Kim's death on the car radio. She thought right then that she could really help the boys. As she told me how she knew she could be good for us, she became quite emotional. My gut feeling about Cara was not wrong. She has been wonderful for them, caring for them and nurturing them in ways I can't. It hasn't been easy for her. Sometimes the boys have given her a rough ride, telling her they wish she'd go away and they want their mummy back. But Cara has stuck it out, understanding what the boys are going through. She has a job with us as long as she wants one. We wouldn't have been able to get through our situation without her. Another good thing about Cara is her boyfriend, Troy Evans. Troy is a top golfer and he's showing me a few tricks on the course.

Today, more than a year after Kim's death, Janey Dopson misses her badly. 'I think about Kim every day, every single day,' she says. 'Things remind me of her. It might be a song that comes on the radio that she loved, or I might walk into my bedroom and I'll see a pair of shoes I bought while she was with me, or when I look at our photos of happy times we shared . . . Before I go to sleep at night I always have a little think about Kim, sometimes I have a bit of a cry.'

Buddy is doing it very tough without Kim. He adored her and she loved him. I've never seen a father and daughter so close. 'I threw in the towel when Kim died. I didn't want to live,' he says. 'I stopped eating for three weeks. I can't spend very long at Kevin and Kim's home because so much there reminds me of her. I have pictures of her in my house but I can't look at them. I sold our family home where she grew up because every time I walked into a room I'd see her there laughing and having fun like she always did. Then Kevin and Wayne and the Broncos gathered around me and told me I had to fight on for the sake of my other children. Wayne was so supportive. He's had heartbreak with his own children and he's been on the brink. He said, "Buddy, you just have to be strong for them." Whenever I see them they can always make me laugh but the problem is I feel so *guilty* laughing, with Kim gone. I shouldn't, because I know she'd want me to carry on. Throughout her illness I was in denial. I refused to let anyone tell me she was sick. I wouldn't listen. Even at Christmas, when Kevin and Kim and the boys were at my house and Kim got sick with a headache and had to go home, I couldn't accept she was seriously ill. I wanted it to go away.

'You have good memories and bad ones. Little things. She was always making me cups of coffee and a sandwich and she'd always take a bite out of my sandwich before giving it to me. Never made a sandwich without doing that. Every Christmas Day Kim and Kevin and the kids would come to my place for one meal and go to Kevin's parents for the other. Even when Kim was so weak she'd still tidy things up around the home. She had a little vacuum cleaner that she would always use. Now Kevin walks around with the vacuum cleaner. Just like Kimmie did. She was a happy person, a straightforward woman who didn't get a big head because she was married to a football star. That's because Kim and Kevin did it tough together for a long time. When they started out they had absolutely nothing. They loved each other and that was that. They fought all the way to get financial stability and when they got there cancer was the reward she got. It's cruel.

'Kim tried to keep her illness from me, and because I was in denial I played along,' Buddy goes on. 'I grew up in the boxing world and always thought I was pretty strong, but I have nowhere near the guts Kim did. How she coped with the disease and the chemotherapy I'll never know. She would come to see me after chemo and she'd smile at me and say, "Hi Dad", as if nothing was wrong. She tried to hide it from me and I found out she rang my sister and said, "This is taking years off Dad's life." As sick as she was, she worried that I couldn't cope. Ten days before she died I went to see her at the hospital. We were sitting there eating and her younger brother Paul's chair broke and he got scratches up his leg. She jumped up and wanted to make him feel better. Soon after that she had a bad turn and had to go back to her room. I said, "I'm not going anywhere. I'll sit here till you feel better." But of course Kim didn't recover. She lingered on for ten more days. I go to the cemetery and I break down every time. It'll never be any other way. I sometimes think it might be easier to bear her death if she'd been a bad person or had done something wrong to me, but she was always beautiful and good. The only consolation is that we loved each other so much.'

CHAPTER TWELVE

# FAREWELLS AND NEW HORIZONS

I talk to Kim all the time. No matter where I am or what I'm doing I take time out for a little chat. She doesn't answer me back in words, but no matter. I earbashed her nonstop all the week leading up to the first State of Origin match in 1998. It was good to be picked in the run-on side for the opening game and I was deadset determined to hang on to my position for all three matches. But first thing's first. In camp for Origin I in Sydney I'd say to Kim: 'Look, you've got to be there. You've got to help us get through this one, because we need you. Bring us luck.' I might be at a movie with the team and I'd drift away and be having a conversation with Kim in my head. I convinced myself that she'd be at that game. There was a song in the charts then, 'The Time of Your Life' by Green

Day. It reminded me of Kim. The song, a catchy ballad, seemed to sum up so many things about her. As we arrived at the Sydney Football Stadium for the match the radio was on in the bus and on came our song. It was like a sign from Kim. 'Oh, Christ,' I thought, 'she's here all right!' I went into that game confident that we wouldn't be beaten, because I knew Kim was upstairs looking after us. It might sound stupid to a lot of people, and I'm no psychic, but I just had this comfortable and confident feeling that we were going to win and I would play well. When the final siren went, with Queensland the victors after I'd set up the winning try with an outrageous speculator kick, I stood and saluted to Kim in heaven. I raised my hand to the sky. It was a sad and happy experience. I was happy that we connected that night at the SFS, but sad that she wasn't really sitting up in the stands.

Last year, 1998, was my best season in rugby league. Seasons 1990, '92 and '97 were good, but '98, the year when the ARL and Super League teams were reunited under the National Rugby League banner, was head and shoulders above them. My only explanation is that losing Kim and being a solo parent made me reassess life, put everything into perspective, and suddenly football wasn't a serious chore to me any more. It was something to *enjoy*. For years I'd fretted that I'd never played to my potential. I was annoyed that for whatever reasons I'd never been able to cement the five-eighth's spot for Queensland and Australia. No matter what I'd achieved, and there have been many highlights in my career, I always found a reason to be dissatisfied. The ordeal with Kim made me realise I wasn't being true to myself, and as soon as I relaxed about my football I became a better player. I thought to myself: 'Bugger it! I'll relax. I'll try not to take football so seriously and go back to the way I was in junior days when I'd do my training, have some fun, show up on match day, go out and give my best and walk off the field with a smile on my face.' That would be my new attitude and it paid dividends in 1998. And instead of worrying about all the top-class young guys challenging for my Broncos and rep teams possie, I relished the pressure they were applying and met it head on. Same thing with the monkey I'd long carried on my back that I wasn't truly a State of Origin standard player, a result of inconsistent selection policies that would see me win the player of the match award one week and be dropped from the side the next. I felt I had been too often made a scapegoat for a Queensland loss. I decided this would be the year when I sent that monkey packing.

I used to get terribly tense before a game. I believed I couldn't play my best unless I was so revved and psyched I was climbing the walls. That's OK once or twice, but you can't sustain that intensity for an entire season, so last year I decided to stay calm through the week, train hard, eat well, enjoy the lead-up to the game. I learned that, if I could manage to do all those things, match day was much easier. These days I'm quiet in the dressing room before a game. I'm confident of my ability, I know what I have to do. If I have to derive strength from outside myself all I have to do is listen to Wayne's wisdom, or look into the eyes of Shane Webcke and Gorden Tallis. Gilly was like that too in the old days. He wouldn't have to say a word to me – just looking into his eyes made me feel capable of anything. In 1998 I soaked up all the premiership, State of Origin and grand final atmosphere, revelled in it, and enjoyed those times more than I ever had. It was no coincidence that, as far as footy went, 1998 was for me as good as it gets.

Origin I, 1998, is considered by many to be among the best – certainly the most exciting – games ever played. It was a wild ride from kickoff to final siren as the lead changed four times. With Lockyer, Sailor, Renouf, Langer and the Smith brothers in Queensland's maroon and New South Wales represented by Brasher, Ettingshausen, Daley, Andrew Johns, Fittler, Harragon and Toovey, the talents of some of the best players of all time exploded all over the paddock that night. Alf's long and short kicking game was pinpoint precise, and we chased his kicks with everything we had. His lethal grubbers brought us our first three tries, Laurie Daley and Adam McDougall mishandling for two of them. Laurie came back at us hard, setting up the Blues' first two tries for Rod Wishart and Tim Brasher and he scored another himself after a frantic scramble on our line. At halftime they were seven points clear, 13–6. We shot back to the lead with tries by Steve Price and Alf, only to be overhauled by four-pointers by Brad Fittler and Steve Menzies. Though opposing the great Daley and a killer defensive back row of Fittler, Nik Kosef and Dean Pay, I made breaks all night. However, it was a kick, not a run, that made that match one I'll never forget.

With 90 seconds left on the clock we were 5 points behind and struggling deep in our territory. 'What the hell,' I thought as the ball shot to me on the first tackle. I reefed that ball upfield. The NSW defence was caught offguard by my kick so early in the tackle count. Ben Ikin, chasing hard, gathered the ball on the first bounce on the halfway line. It went to Darren Smith, to Tonie Carroll who crashed over for a try. One point behind with the conversion to come. As the siren rang, Darren Lockyer kicked the goal. Queensland 24 – NSW 23. In the exultant celebrations that followed the miracle win, I thought of my team-mates, my brothers and family. I thought of my sons. I thought of my conversations with Kim and saluted the stars.

Laurie killed us in Origin II at Suncorp Stadium. He inspired the Blues to a 26–10 win and so set up an epic decider at the Sydney Football Stadium. In Origin III, everything clicked for us from the kickoff. In the opening minutes, Wendell Sailor, who all week had been the target of accusations that he was shaky under the high ball, defused a bomb and sped 40 metres upfield. Building on his break, we moved the ball. It passed through seven sets of hands before I backed up to score in the seventh minute. This time there was no comeback from the Blues. Gorden Tallis, Shane Webcke, Darren and Jason Smith had the measure of the NSW forwards, with Gorden having one of his great tearaway games. Fittingly, the final try was a Langer special. He got the ball close to the NSW line and shaped as if he was going to kick. The defence hung off. Instead, Alf ran the ball and scored a try untouched. The final score was a decisive 19–4. Origin III, and the series, was ours. It was our first series win since 1995. Victory was so sweet, and my strong form throughout the three classic games erased once and for all any fears I had that I could not cut it at this most demanding and unforgiving level of rugby league.

In the dressing room afterwards I was near tears. I couldn't remember ever feeling better about a game of football. There was something strange about Origin III, an eerie expectation that things would work out great. I felt so good when I ran onto the field. I felt totally satisfied about the way I played and my contribution to our win. Before the match, Jack and Billy asked me to score a try. The try I scored that night was really special because it meant so much to Queensland and the team, but I also sent a thought home to Jack when I slid over. I said to myself as I was engulfed by joyful team-mates: 'They'll like that back home.' I had a chat to Kim before that game, too. Origin III was for her. She was crazy about State of Origin. She knew how much the games mean to me and how I wanted so much to play well. I'm sure she was there celebrating with us that night.

For the first time ever, too, Brisbane won the premiership in the same year that Queensland, loaded with 12 Broncos, took out the State of Origin. This was some achievement when you consider the competing demands of both. And of course, making 1998 one of the most gruelling rep seasons ever, there was the Test series against New Zealand with Darren Lockyer, Wendell Sailor, Steve Renouf, Brad Thorn, Gorden Tallis, Darren Smith, Alf Langer, Shane Webcke and me getting the call to play for our country, and Wayne was the coach. In the domestic comp, the Broncos rewrote the record books. Our 149 tries was the most ever scored in a season; as were our total points (812). Our 54-point winning margins over Norths and North Queensland were our highest ever. The 38 points we racked up against Canterbury in the grand final was the highest score in a premiership decider ever and our winning margin of 26 points was also the biggest.

I started the year in good form and my purple patch lasted all season. Looking back, it seems like a dream, a season of red letter days. In *Rugby League 1999*, the NRL's official yearbook, editor David Middleton summed up my season this way:

> The contribution of five-eighth Kevin Walters was significant to the Broncos' success in 1998. The popular Queensland and Australian representative lost his wife to cancer early in the year, but his ability to rise above the tragedy was a source of inspiration for the club. Walters was a key figure in many of the Broncos' triumphs and enjoyed his finest season at representative level. He was instrumental in Queensland's dramatic last-ditch win in the first State of Origin match, and played his way back into the Australian Test side after an absence of five years.

Things on the field that I once found hard came to me easily. My attack, defence and kicking games, possibly for the reasons I mentioned earlier, were never better than in 1998, and I was able to maintain my form. I was happy with my combination with Alf (Tony Durkin wrote that 'without Walters outside him, Langer is like a horse without a jockey'), and with my service to my outside flyers Renouf, Darren Smith, Hancock, Devere, Carroll and Sailor, who scored plenty of tries and comprised the best three-quarter line in the game, and Darren Lockyer, who chimed on to my passes from fullback.

My watershed year has given me some great memories. I remember marking Anthony Mundine, now back at St George, at Kogarah Oval and winning a points decision. We whacked Saints 30–18 in spite of fierce barracking from the unforgiving locals. Gorden Tallis really copped it that afternoon from supporters of his former club who sledged him and pelted tennis balls at him. 'Tallis Spells Scum' read one sign in the outer. It was extremely satisfying for him – and for me too – when he sealed the match for us with a powerful surge through four defenders to score the final try. Against Norths at ANZ, Alf and I combined as well as we ever have in our 60–6 victory. Our 26–6 defeat of 1997 ARL premiers Newcastle at their homeground Marathon Stadium was important because it proved we were the best side, ARL or Super League.

That season saw the coming of age of some hot young Broncos, ensuring that Queensland and Australian sides will be rich in skill and toughness for a decade to come. There is Tallis the firebrand, a brutally uncompromising player who has still only scratched the surface of his potential. It has taken time for Gorden to adapt to our style at the Broncos. 'I'm still coming to terms with the control the likes of Allan Langer and Kevin Walters have over a game,' he has said. Wayne Bennett said of the young international: 'Gorden feels he has to lead from the front and be involved all the time. As a footballer he is just so raw, and there is a lot of ability underneath the surface that is about to explode. He is one of the rare breed who hurts you when he carries the football, and that is a fearsome quality.' When Gorden was starting his career with us, Tony Durkin of *Rugby League Week* asked me how I thought he would go. 'Gorden will be our new Gilly,' I said. 'You need a bloke like him, someone who will plant fear into the opposition. It's a bit like having a big German shepherd sitting at your front gate.' We'd heard how other forward packs turned it up when playing against him, so short was his fuse, and even at training he was dangerous. 'He'll deadset kill someone soon,' I said. 'He has all this anger inside him just bursting to get out, and we hope he gets to release it in a game – for us.'

Darren Lockyer confirmed his promise as the best fullback in rugby league. He's a future Broncos captain. He is richly talented, a beautiful, lightning-quick runner with the ball and a nerveless kicker. He can tackle and takes the high ball fearlessly. He is level-headed too, as shown by the way he put his nightmare game against New Zealand in 1997 behind him and went on to great heights. Shane Webcke has also entrenched himself in the Queensland and Australian teams. He's a country boy who owns land at Leyburn. When he arrived at the Broncos, Shane weighed 120kg but Wayne knocked him into condition and he's now shaping as the new Glenn Lazarus, tight, tough and a good man for a crisis. Throw in our classy young players Ben Walker, Petero Civoniceva, Tonie Carroll and Brad Thorn and established stars Peter Ryan, Wendell Sailor and Steve Renouf and you just know there will be life in the Broncos long after old blokes like me have hung up their boots.

About three weeks out from the grand final against the Canterbury Bulldogs I did something I never thought I'd do. I went to see a psychic. I needed to make some kind of contact with Kim. I'm not sure what was happening, but I think I did make contact. I sent my love to her through the psychic. The psychic, whom I'd never met before, astounded me. She knew that Kim was a fussy gardener who hated weeds and that Jack was having trouble holding his pen at school. There were many other things she knew about us. I asked her whether there was anything I could do to help Buddy Facer, who was – and still is – doing it tough over Kim. The psychic said: 'No, Kim's father sees things in black and white.' That's exactly how he is. I was deadset sure she was talking with Kim's spirit. At the end of the session I asked the psychic whether Brisbane would win the grand final. I know this sounds crazy, but the psychic replied: 'Yes, you'll win, but there's a guy in your team who needs to lift his game a bit. He's not quite playing to the best of his ability at the moment but, if he can, you guys are going to win. You know who that player is.' I did. It was Alf. Not that he was playing badly, just not quite up to his usual incredibly high standard. As it happened, Alf turned up a gear in the big one and we won. I'll go back and see that psychic again. It's just so comforting to believe that Kim is out there somewhere looking over us. A wonderful and reassuring thought. I'm sure Kim is at our house all the time. I can feel her. I'm certain she was with us on Jack's birthday. I like to think so, anyway. It helps me cope.

Our upset 15–10 loss to Parramatta in the second quarter-final qualifier, our first game in the eight-team finals series, knocked any complacency out of us. The defeat was a severe embarrassment, for we were everyone's premiership favourite. It ensured that we were well and truly psyched and focused when we met Melbourne Storm in the second elimination semi. Our forwards ripped into the premiership newcomers, who seemed shocked by our ferocity. A number of commentators reckoned that we seemed unusually aggressive against Melbourne – one used the word 'nasty'. The Storm's hot young halves Brett Kimmorley and Scott Hill were on the back foot from the outset as their forwards buckled in the trenches. In fairness to Kimmorley, he was groggy after copping a high tackle from Peter Ryan that led to Peter being outed for three weeks and missing the grand final. Kimmorley made uncharacteristic errors, kicking into touch on the full twice, and missing a tackle on me that led to a try. We scored six tries to one in our 30–6 victory. I won man of the match, *Rugby League Week* summing up: 'Broncos five-eighth Kevin Walters has had his best-ever season. He drove Storm lock Tawera Nikau to distraction with his footwork.' Next up were the Sydney City Roosters in the first grand final qualifier. That day, at ANZ, we were ready to rumble. At the final siren we'd plucked the Roosters 46–18. Darren Lockyer was irresistible. He scored three tries and four goals in the game.

Wayne had prepared us like a champion racehorse and by the time we ran onto the field to meet Canterbury in the grand final, we were champing at the bit. The Bulldogs, as we knew they would, hit us with everything in the first half and led 12–10 at the break. We didn't panic, knowing that if we played to our ability all would be well. Sure enough, right after halftime, Tonie Carroll, Wendell and Gorden had scored powerhouse tries and we led 26–12. We ran Canterbury ragged and scored another two tries – to Phillip Lee and Darren Smith in his last game for us before joining Canterbury for 1999. Typical of our determination that day was when I kicked deep into Bulldog territory and chased hard with three or four other Broncos right with me. We cornered their winger Daryl Halligan who'd retrieved the kick and picked him up and carried him back over his line. We scored from the resulting goal line dropout. 'The Broncos would hold their heads up in any era, against any team,' Bulldogs coach Steve Folkes generously declared. Wayne said: 'This team did everything they could possibly achieve. We have never won a premiership the same year Queensland have won an Origin series, and we also finished minor premiers. It wasn't possible for this team to achieve any more. It was a real team effort.' Wayne refused to be drawn into comparisons with our 1992 and 1993 premiership-winning teams. I won't buy into that either, but I will say that our performances throughout 1998 established us as one of the all-time great club teams.

There were nine of us selected in the Australian squad to meet the Kiwis at Suncorp Stadium on 9 October: Lockyer, Renouf, Sailor, Smith, Langer, Tallis, Webcke, Thorn and me. Alf was skipper, Wayne was our coach. It was a proud feeling to be in the run-on side for this revenge Test. The Kiwis were one-up in the series, having towelled us 22–16 back in April. We had to win to keep the three-Test series alive. It was my first game for Australia since the 1994 Kangaroo tour and my first Test since 1992's World Cup final against England. I had made myself unavailable for the Australian Super League side that toured England in November the year before. Kim, in the final ravaging stages of her illness, needed me desperately then, and so did our boys, and anyway I would not have been able to bear being away from them.

Now, with Laurie Daley and Brad Fittler injured, I knew I was a chance to make the Test side which was picked after the 1998 grand final, but my heart wasn't in it at first. I saw Wayne and ruled myself out of contention. It had been a long season and I had spent many nights away from the boys. I figured my job for the Broncos and Queensland was done, and that enough was enough. Wayne, however, talked me around, convincing me that my country needed me. So I played in the Brisbane international and went to New Zealand for the Third Test but had to pull out with a torn hamstring, so I returned home to the boys immediately and watched the Test on TV.

The Kiwis' game plan in the match I played was painfully obvious from the opening whistle. New Zealand hit us with everything. Steve Price and Steve Renouf were knocked out by high shots, and Shane Webcke and Robbie Kearns had head wounds that required stitching. By and large, we refused to get sucked in, although of course Gorden, who scored two tries in an inspiring performance, had his moments. Alf calls Gorden 'The Kettle', because he blows off so much steam. What an exciting player. I've never seen a more dominant performance from a forward than his in that Test against New Zealand. Without Gorden, I don't think we would have won the game. He met their aggression with some of his own. He was the one who revved us up and gave it to the Kiwis straight: 'Righto, you —! I'm gonna give you some back!' When we saw him knocking them backwards we got behind him. At the end of the game the score was Australia 30 – New Zealand 12. All Australia's tries were scored by Broncos: Tallis, Lockyer, Thorn and me.

Then we won the Third Test – without me – 36–16. At the end of the game, Jason Smith was interviewed on television and said: 'Kevvie, this one's for you!' I appreciated being remembered so much. On and off the field, Jason is a class act. I would love to have played club football with Jason. We combine well together.

At the end of the football year, I was a satisfied man. My club, my State and my country had all been victorious, and I was proud of the part I played. But until the start of the new season in 1999, the only games that mattered would be the ones I played with Jack, Billy and Jett.

As I write this book, in mid-1999, it's looking as if the Broncos will have their work cut out winning a third grand final in a row. We had a horror start to the year, losing match after match, and in May we were coming stone last in the comp. Looking back at our early results this year is a nightmarish experience. Put it all down to our complacent attitude. If your attitude is not right it shows up in defence. Bad attitude is not so damaging in attack because it's easy to get the football and run with it, but nobody enjoys tackling too much. The boys weren't committed to getting up and doing the extra little things in defence for each other. At the Broncos we have a thing where our defence is broken up into three teams defending the left side, the ruck, and right side, and this year our defensive errors have been up in all areas. In 1998 when things were going well for us, our worst defensive performance in any area would be 15–20 defensive errors in a match, and our best less than 10. This year we've been making 25-plus errors a game. That means points against you. Our attack is fine, and we're scoring as heavily as in 1998, but our opponents have been scoring more.

In our eleven-year history, we had never lost the opening game of the season, but this year, in a warning of worse to come, Canberra beat us 28–20 after Ben Walker was sent off for a swinging arm and I had to leave the field with a pinched nerve in my hip. We were rusty, our timing was off and we slipped off tackles. Physio through the week got me back on the field against Cronulla the following week, but in a patchy, scrappy game at ANZ Stadium, we lost again, 14–6. Fans waiting for one of our trademark comebacks after the Sharks led us by 4 at halftime waited . . . and waited, and went home disappointed. What had come together naturally for us in the past – a whirlwind 16 points or so to turn defeat into victory – just didn't happen. When Melbourne Storm thrashed us 48–6 at ANZ in Round 3, it was the worst defeat in our history. They scored eight tries to one. We dropped the ball, threw loose passes, missed tackles. We were bloody disgraceful.

We were better against Cronulla the next week, scoring three tries to the Sharks' three, but when you're down you're down, and we lost again, 20–18. It was Canterbury's turn to beat us in Round 5, 20–16. Once again, in a promising sign, we scored as many tries as our opposition. It hurt that the man of the match was our much-missed old team-mate Darren Smith. Five losses on the trot, equalling our worst losing run ever, in 1989, when we lost five on the run and missed the semis. Most of the games we've lost this season have been there to be won, but we couldn't pull off a victory. And you get the same number of points for a 2-point loss as you do for a 20-point thrashing: none. Certainly injuries disrupted our combination and left us understrength. At various times in the first 10 rounds of the comp Michael Hancock, Peter Ryan, Steve Renouf, Michael Devere, Gorden Tallis and Darren Lockyer were out injured. That, however, didn't stop us in past years.

At last, in Round 6 against South Sydney, a win! It all came back, passes stuck, tackles were made, luck ran our way. We walloped the Rabbitohs 30–10. Shane Webcke, Gorden Tallis, Petero Civoniceva, Brad Thorn, Kevin Campion and Andrew Gee outmuscled the Souths forwards and suddenly Alf and I had the room to move we'd lacked all year. That was the game when the Rabbitohs' halfback Tricky Trindall sledged Alf viciously, calling him old and broken down. Alf seemed to laugh it off. We hoped we were back on track, but our high hopes lasted just one week, until we lost 19–18 to the Newcastle Knights. Once more we scored the same number of tries as the victors. We played well that day, and five Broncos were picked in the Australian side that night: Alf, Gorden Tallis, Shane Webcke, Darren Lockyer and Wendell Sailor. Our lock Kevin 'Champion' Campion had a blinder. Nine minutes from fulltime he put me into a gap and all of a sudden I was 20 years old again and running in the open. I passed to hooker Luke Priddis, who scored. Lockyer converted and it was 18–18. But three minutes later Matthew Johns kicked a field goal and the defeat was demoralising. The following week, just when we thought we were turning the corner, we had a shocker against North Queensland and could only salvage a 20–20 draw. It was a miserable performance. Ben Walker replaced Alf in the second half. When Wayne Bennett gave Alf the hook and he trudged off the field none of us realised he'd never play again.

In the shower after the match I went up to Alf with a big grin on my face and yelled: 'Hey, Alf, show us the red mark around your neck from getting the old shepherd's hook!' He looked at me hard and snapped: 'They'll never do that to me again. That will never happen again.' I said: 'What do you mean?' He just remarked quietly: 'I'm retiring.' I said, 'Oh yeah, right,' and left him alone. That night we went out for a few drinks and Alf was more emotional than I'd ever seen him. He is a proud man and being replaced hurt him badly. He said he was determined to retire. He told me he loved me. I said, trying to lighten the situation: 'What! Alf you've never stopped bagging me!' He said: 'I've made my mind up, Kevvie. I'm never playing again.' I came back at him: 'Alf, stand down from the team for two weeks, train but don't play, and see if you miss it.' But when Alf makes his mind up that's it. Back at the hotel he phoned his wife Janine and broke the news to her. Next morning he told Wayne and the press conference announcing the sad news was called.

After the press conference, Wayne pulled me aside and told me I would be the Broncos' new captain. My first game as skipper was against the Storm in

Melbourne. We played that game for Alf, but in the end that made no difference because we were beaten 28–18. I felt I had my best game of the season. It sure was different without Alf. After 10 years playing together it was strange to be partnering Ben Walker, a rep star of the future but a young man with big boots to fill. If he was feeling the pressure of replacing a legend, Ben, a cool young man who I love to bet with on the result of Friday night footy games on TV, was not showing it. He told me after the game: 'I didn't feel any pressure from the club and I didn't put any on myself. I was caught up in all the media hype about Alf's retirement during the week, so I didn't even really think about the match until it was time to play. It's impossible for me to emulate Alf's feats, so I'll just be playing my own game. Alf didn't give me any advice. He's a man of few words and about two minutes before kickoff against Melbourne he wished me all the best. That was it.'

Before kickoff against the very hot Sydney City Roosters at ANZ in Round 10, Broncos fans had a chance to farewell Alf. Celebrities and former Broncos stars clapped Alfie as he walked, in his civvies, onto the field. Lord Mayor Jim Soorley presented him with the keys of the city of Brisbane. Alf then made a slow lap of honour in a car around the stadium. He kept jumping out to shake fans' hands and get hugs from tearful supporters. One last wave to the crowd and he was off up the tunnel, the lump in his throat the size of a pumpkin.

We lost 26–16 but, with stronger performances by

Tonie Carroll, Michael Hancock and a confident showing by Ben Walker, the signs were there that our game was at last falling into place. Lote Tuqiri gave glimpses of his wonderful promise. In the 64th minute, we turned on a Broncos special. I put Phil Lee into a gap, he shot the ball to Benny Walker who, Renouf-style, upped a gear and glided around Roosters fullback Andrew Walker to score. Just 15 minutes to go and we were down just 4 points, 20–16. Unfortunately, our handling errors allowed Sydney back into the game. Another try to them and we were history yet again.

It's too early to say yet, and no one is getting carried away, but the Roosters match may have been a turning point. By then, all the young Broncos who'd been thrown into first grade a year too early, because of our injury toll, were gaining confidence. Shaun Berrigan, Lote Tuqiri, Dane Carlaw, Brad Myers and the Walker brothers are the Broncos' future.

The next week we beat Balmain in front of a parochial home crowd at Leichhardt, then a bye gave us two more points and a chance to lick our wounds. With Gorden, Steve Renouf and Darren Lockyer back in the side we smashed Wests 50–0 in Round 13. I had my best game of the year and I felt my scrumbase combination with Ben Walker coming together. Then we kept the powerful Penrith Panthers pointless in a 28–0 walloping at ANZ. Suddenly, we were just a few points out of the top eight. But, as Wayne kept drumming into us then, if we're still travelling as well as now in 10 weeks, we'll start thinking about semi-finals.

I got picked for State of Origin again. I thought I might have been captain with Alf out of the equation, but Adrian Lam got the job. I understand there was a feeling among some selectors that I should have been overlooked altogether. Nothing changes! Whatever, we won 9–8 with Mat Rogers getting all our points in a gruelling game, and I was very happy with how I played, especially in defence. My hit on Nik Kosef that saw the ball explode from the tackle was satisfying. Jason Hetherington at hooker played a blinder, and all of the Broncos lifted their game.

For Origin II, Adrian was injured and I led the Maroons against New South Wales at Stadium Australia in front of nearly 90,000 parochial Blues fans who braved driving rain that fell the entire game. We had a horror start when the Blues moved the ball wide in the opening seconds, Andrew Johns to Laurie Daley to Ryan Girdler, who raced into the clear then passed to Robbie Ross who sprinted 40 metres to the line. Less than a minute into the game we were down 6–0. All that mattered to me then was to settle my team down and make sure they kept their heads up. We hung in there. After 20 minutes they hadn't scored again and we'd crept up to 6–2. I knew there would be no opening of the floodgates. The forward exchanges were brutal. Jason Hetherington, playing another fine game, and Shane Webcke gangtackled a rampaging Mark Carroll and knocked Spud out. Gorden Tallis looked further afield to create a little mayhem and came to grips with NSW centre Terry Hill. After 25 minutes we were attacking on their 20-metre line. I got the ball, dummied left, straightened and threw a face ball – a carbon copy of the pass that sent Steve Renouf over in the World Cup final seven years before – which put Jason Smith into a gap. He sent to Mat Rogers who tore over for a try. With the conversion it was 8–6 to us. Just before halftime, referee Steven Clark ruled that our fullback Robbie O'Davis had knocked on when it looked for all the world that he'd fumbled the ball backwards. A couple of rucks later, Laurie powered over near the posts. It was 12–8 to NSW at halftime, and that remained the score at the final siren. But I was again very happy with my game. My defence was sound, and I felt good with the ball in my hands. One critic summed up my performance: 'Led the Maroons well and was instrumental in their lone try. Still a force at this elite level.'

We were disappointed not to wrap up the series 2–0 in Sydney, but the feeling in our camp after the game was 'Bring on Origin III in Brisbane to decide matters'. Before the game I was asked whether being Queensland captain meant much to me. Of course it did, it meant plenty, but after all these years, after all the ups and downs, I knew it would mean a lot more if we were to win the series.

In the event Adrian Lam was again captain for Origin III and I was happy with that. At any rate, it was academic because hamstring injury prevented me from playing and I watched the 10-all draw from the sideline.

I'm 32 now, in 1999, and after 13 seasons in first grade, 11 Tests for Australia and more than 20 State of

Origin matches my career is winding down. I've signed with the Broncos for the 2000 season and after that I'll see what happens. I might coach, but coaching is a long, long road. You have to start from scratch, build yourself up over a three or four year period with a minor side before you're ready to take on a first grade outfit. I would really enjoy being a coach, and it would give me great satisfaction. If you're being paid for doing a job you love you're very lucky. I don't think I'd ever go back to being a carpenter fulltime, but if I had to I certainly would.

More likely I'll try to get involved in media work. I do segments and interviews on TV when invited, and have managed to keep my nose clean since the John Quayle stuff-up. I've got a footy gig as Brisbane correspondent on Optus Vision's Tuesday night 'Winners' show with Roy Masters, Terry Kennedy and Brad Clyde and I do spots on Triple M radio's 'Blood, Sweat 'n' Beers'. On Mondays and Fridays the station's Morning Crew rings me to chat on air about the game. I write a couple of columns for rural Queensland papers. Being on TV has never bothered me. I'm never likely to suffer from stagefright. I like to work ad lib, rather than with a script. I'm always comfy raving on about footy. I love it, it's my industry. I don't see it as work but as fun.

When Kim died I had two choices: be strong the way she wanted me to be and do the best for our sons and myself, or fall apart with self-pity and bawl my eyes out every day. I promised Kim I'd never fall apart because that's the soft option. Besides, with my family and footy now and all the challenges that lie ahead there's too much going on in my life. I'm proud of the way I've handled things since we lost Kim. I never look for sympathy. We have lost a wife and mother, but we have each other and a treasure trove of loving memories that will keep us strong throughout whatever the future brings.

My grandad, Harold Hill, who had been very supportive of my career, passed away on 21 June 1999 – the Monday before Origin III. Kim's tragedy – and Grandad's passing away – has, if anything, brought my parents and family even closer together. I take the boys to Ipswich every chance I get. Jack plays five-eighth with my old team, Booval Swifts, and I drive him out to training on Wednesday nights. We drop in on Mum and Dad and Mum will have one of her special roasts in the oven and there'll be one or two or three of my brothers with their kids and there'll be a backyard footy game. After my brothers and I grew up and left home, Dad put up a greenhouse where we used to play. But today there is a new generation of Walters kids, the children of my brothers, who are just as mad-keen on football as we were. So Dad had no choice. He pulled that greenhouse down, regrassed the lawn and rigged up the old floodlight again.

Once again, epic matches are contested into the night. Once again, there are great tries scored and tackles made. Once again, there are tears and tantrums as the kids get stuck in. Sometimes Steve, Andrew, Brett and I join in for old times' sake. Dad and Mum referee as they always did. Mum has her hose handy. Dad's there on his step, like in the old days, although he's given up the smokes and he's as likely to be swigging on a Diet Coke as having a beer.

And crashtackling your brother onto the concrete path still brings an automatic penalty.

# AFTERWORDS

## *Family, friends and footballers on Kevin Walters' life and career*

BRAD FITTLER

On his day, I rate Kevin the best five-eighth in the world. When Brisbane are going forward, Kevin has been a real handful running off Alfie. He does everything superbly – sets up play, he is always there in support and he runs with the ball in front of him, which keeps the opposition defence in two minds. Kevin has continued to get better each year, and the 1998 season was the best I have seen him play. He absolutely brained them and showed why he's such a class act.

I put Kevin in the same category as Terry Lamb.

Someone who wasn't able to cement a spot in the Australian side, but without peer when it comes to club football. I consider that to be an even bigger wrap, because, like Terry, Kevin has consistently performed week in and week out over a number of years. I can tell you it takes a player of real quality to do that. Kevin amazes me with his energy level, and you can tell from his body language that he loves his footy. Kevin and Alfie were the masterminds behind Brisbane's dominance during the 1990s, and as long as they were together as a combination the Broncos were a specially formidable outfit.

Kevin may come across as just a clown, but he takes his football seriously. When it is time to train, he always gives 100 per cent and never shirks it. No one in football circles has a bad word to say about Kevin – that shows the quality of the bloke. I love being around him because he always makes you laugh and have a good time. Kevin doesn't have to bung things on, his humour comes naturally, which makes him even funnier.

I had a great friend who died, so I know how tough losing someone who's close can be. But I have never lost a wife, so I can't imagine what Kevin has been through. To be able to put everything to one side and play sensational football, as he did and is still doing, just shows the courage of the bloke.

WALLY LEWIS

The greatest game Kevin has ever played has been staying solid in the tough times when Kim was ill and then after she passed away. People were waiting for him to crack, but he couldn't afford to buckle. He could have collapsed and gone into a deep depression, but he couldn't risk the welfare of his three young kids. He had to stay standing for their sake, and this example will help them with their growing up.

No one can imagine the torment he was going through with Kim, but to keep performing the way he did just shows the character of the bloke. Time became Kevin's closest ally. He knew the inevitable was going to happen, which I suppose gave him a little bit more scope to deal with the situation.

Kevin has a strong spirit. He is a wonderful joker. He reminds me of a kid in Grade 5. He tells these stupid jokes with a silly smirk on his face. But the great thing about Kevin is that he can always make you laugh, no matter what the situation. Kevin would always say to me, 'How are you going, King?', which would drive me mad. At times, he can be a dickhead, but I say that in the nicest possible way.

I remember when we were in a camp in Sydney and this Chinese bloke came up to me. When he said, 'You're King Wally', his accent made it come out as 'Ling Wally'. Kevin and Alf were standing nearby and really gave it to me from then on. Whether we were in the lift or at training, the pair would constantly repeat: 'Ling Wally, Ling Wally.' Even now when they see me they say it!

What I really admire about Kevin is the fact that he can switch off from football, something I was unable to do. That's helped his longevity in the game.

His form in the 1998 Origin series was superb. I don't think he could erase his bad memories of previous series, but I know his efforts last year would have given him great pleasure. As an Origin player, I think he has become more streetwise after so many disappointments. Certainly no one would have begrudged him his moment in the sun.

LAURIE DALEY

As a player, when I come up against Brad Fittler or Matthew Johns I know I have to raise the level of my game. I put Kevin in that same category. He is stronger than you think and often he's put me on my backside. I regard Kevin as a priceless footballer. He can play anywhere in the backs and forwards, and his presence around a football club is invaluable. Kevin is difficult to play against for a number of reasons. Before a game, I don't talk to him, but I may acknowledge him with a wink. I'm pumped up and have a serious expression on my face, then I look up and see Kevin laughing at me. It can be very offputting, but that's Kevin.

Every football club needs a bloke like Kevin. No matter what the situation, he has the ability to make you laugh. He is someone everyone loves being around. There's nothing false about him. He's a genuine bloke. He is always trying to take the piss out of you, and when he teamed up with Alf it was always a laugh a minute.

I think most people would have thought Kevin's football would suffer after Kim's death, but in fact I reckon he had his best season in 1998. I was disappointed New South Wales lost the Origin series, but I was happy for Kevin because of all the pain he had gone through. In the past he was blamed for Queensland's defeats, but in 1998 he proved to many that he was a champion.

As for the Broncos, Kevin has played an enormous role in the side's dominance throughout the 1990s. He is a senior figure, a team leader and a great role model for the younger players.

BEN ELIAS

When you're in trouble, you look to someone like Kevin to get you out of that hole. Over the years, when the Broncos have needed a piece of brilliance he has provided it. This is the sign of a class player. Kevin has done everything in the game, won premierships, played State of Origin football and Tests. He has left a significant mark on the Broncos.

I can't imagine what he went through losing Kim, but to be on top of his game like he was in 1998 is testimony to the courage of the bloke. He showed true champion qualities and I have nothing but admiration for him.

As a practical joker, I regard Kevin as a genius. I thought I was a big gee-up artist, but Kevin puts me to shame. He is a court jester and is clever with words. No one was safe from Kevin's practical jokes, and I can tell you Keith Barnes, our team manager on the 1990 Kangaroo tour, was happy to see the back of him. Following our First Test loss at Wembley, there was a bit of gloom and doom in the camp, but it was Kevin who helped lift the morale in the side. He organised a game of cricket in our hotel corridor, using a snooker cue as a bat, snooker balls as cricket balls, and a sheet of glass for the wicket. Understandably, the batsmen were desperate not to get out. At the end of the match, there was broken glass everywhere and the players had to fork out for the repairs, but no one cared because we had so much fun. I think that game brought everyone in the team closer together. We refocused to win the last two Tests and retain the Ashes. Kevin can take some of the credit for that.

BRAD IZZARD

I regard Laurie Daley as the best five-eighth in the world, but Kevin is not far behind him. He has all the skills and has thrived playing behind Brisbane's superb forward pack. He reminds me a lot of Terry Lamb because, when there's half a break made, Kevin's there backing up.

Kevin's wife wouldn't have wanted him to fold after she died, so knowing that would have been a huge motivational factor for him in 1998. He would have been playing on adrenalin all season. But it showed the courage of the man to put this dreadful tragedy in the background and play sensational football. Kim would have been proud of him, and you can't help but feel happy for Kevin that footballing-wise he had such a great season.

TONY DURKIN

As editor of *Rugby League Week*, I've reported on Kevin's career now for more than 13 years. So I can say that, when the time comes for Kevvie to knock on the front door of the home for retired footballers, he'll leave some memories behind. Father of three young boys, coping so courageously after the loss of Kim. The wag of Queensland's *Footy Show* and myriad other media performances. One of the most talented rugby league players of the past decade.

Who can forget the brilliant pass to a flying Steve Renouf for Australia's winning try in the 1992 World Cup final at Wembley? Or his visionary kick in the dying stages of Origin I in 1998 that led to a last-minute try and a Queensland victory.

Then, of course, there was his contribution to the Broncos. As junior partner in the Alf and Kevvie show, Walters was the perfect foil. While opposing defences kept suffocating tabs on the brilliant Langer, his five-eighth monotonously gave them the slip. The pair first teamed for the Broncos in 1990 and it is no fluke that in the following eight seasons they won four premierships and a World Club Championship. Other top scrumbase combinations came and went in that period, but few were able to dominate like the Broncos pairing. In football's pecking order, Langer was always a skerrick ahead of Walters, and Kevvie knew that. But he never minded playing second fiddle to his mate from Ipswich, and was not offended when Wayne Bennett appointed Alfie captain of the Broncos in 1992 – ahead of the next best candidate,

Kevvie. Kevin was never envious of Alf's standing in the game.

What did wound him, though, was the shoddy treatment he received over the years from the Queensland State of Origin selectors. Rugby league supporters far and wide rated him with the elite players, but it seemed that some very influential people in his own backyard harboured doubts about him. Of the 22 matches he's played to date for the Maroons, nine have been from the bench. Even in the 1999 series, with Langer out of the picture after his sudden retirement, Walters' inclusion in the Queensland side was far from a unanimous decision, and astonishingly he was overlooked as captain for the first game, only being given the much deserved honour when Adrian Lam was unfit for the second match. But in the 1999 series, as he has always done before, he proved his knockers wrong.

KATHRYN McKEWIN

As business programs manager of the Wesley Hospital, I've had a lot to do with Kevin since the Kim Walters Choices Program was established in March 1998. To me he is not a huge, commanding personality, but a genuine, no-frills man who instils confidence. If Kevin says something, he means it. If he undertakes to do something, he'll do it. There is an honesty about him that people pick up on. I go all goosy thinking about the way he's touched the lives of so many people. There was a man, aged 90, in intensive care who had been a sportsman in his day. I introduced him to

Kevvie. 'You'd be a Walters, wouldn't you!' the old guy said. Kevvie made him feel so special. He'd drop in on the man in his ward. I was conscious that Kim had died just two floors above and I said to Kevin, 'Do you have a problem coming here?', and he just replied, 'No, no, it's fine.'

What sums up Kevin Walters better than anything is when I introduced him to a woman who was suffering with breast cancer and he asked about her husband. 'Will he cope?' he wanted to know. 'Is he a good man?' Such things are important to Kevin.

SANDRA WALTERS

I'm his Mum, so you wouldn't expect me to say bad things about him, but Kevin has been a wonderful son. My memories? I can still see him as a kid bawling in the yard when he was losing a footy match. Then he'd run inside and paint a different team's colour on his T-shirt and go out there and start again. I can see him in his school uniform and I'd say, 'Where are you going?', and he'd reply, 'I'm off to see my bird, Kim.' And the superstition about the roast. Every time the Broncos won I'd have to cook a roast. Over the years I got so sick of roasts when they were winning game after game. Early this season, 1999, wins – and roasts – were rare, so I guess these days we're enjoying a little more variety in our meals. And also I'll never forget Kevin putting Steve Renouf over for the winning try against Great Britain in the 1992 World Cup final at Wembley. That and the Broncos grand final wins would have to be the greatest memories. Another thing I'll never forget is when Kevin waved to Kimmie up in the heavens after the first State of Origin game in 1998.

Kevin has always been a bit of a comedian, and it's good today to see him beginning to smile again. While Kim was sick he wasn't cracking too many jokes, but the jokes are starting to come out again.

Today his life is going on. Kevin has got to pick himself up, start a new chapter in his life. He's still so young, and there's still such a long way to go.

With Kevin, Kerrod and Steve now at or nearing the end of their careers, I'm getting used to the fact that my own life as a football mother is about to end. No more getting worked up and wanting to run onto the field when my sons get hurt, no more abusing selectors and coaches! Now I'll have to get used to being a football grandmother – because, of KG's and my eleven grandkids, eight are boys and they're all into their footy. Like their dads did, they play for Booval Swifts down the street. Kevin's Jack has a bit of size about him and scores plenty of tries. I'd be disappointed if they didn't play, but it wouldn't be the end of the world. Rugby league is different today to how it used to be. It's more skilful, but there's so much pressure since the big money came into the game.

All in all, football has been good to our family. So many great times, so many friends. KG and I are proud to have had three sons play rugby league for their country. Our family has had its ups and downs, like any family, but we stick together and we get through.